Words Unspoken

The Science, Experience, and Treatment of Stuttering

Tom Lovett

First edition May 2023

Edited by Steffannie Alter
Cover Design by Jackie Jack *iamjackiejack.com*

ISBN 979-8-9880699-0-4 (paperback)
ISBN 979-8-9880699-1-1 (digital)

Published by Ingram Spark

tomlovett.com

Contact: hi@tomlovett.com
Distributors: wholesale@tomlovett.com

Table of Contents

Preface

On January 12, 2018, I realized that I needed to do something about stuttering. The night before, I had read yet another post on a stuttering forum from a person who felt they were drowning under the weight of their stutter. I had commented on a few of these posts, sharing advice that I had gained from my experience, or letting them know that I, too, had once been in that same darkness but it was possible to make it out.

I only responded to a small number of these posts, though. I felt like it wasn't practical to spend hours of my life writing something that would only be seen by a handful of people before disappearing below the scroll line. And anyways, a fresh post just like it would surely appear a few days later.

I felt guilty, though. Given the frequency of these posts, there was clearly a larger problem at hand and I wasn't doing everything I could to help. But this particular post was so poignant that it lingered in the back of my mind the following day.

I was weighed down by struggles of my own at the time too: I had recently been fired from my first software job and the subsequent job hunt was not going well. In addition to that, my family was in the middle of a bitter fight. (And to top it off, it was another cold, gray, and miserable Boston winter.)

That day, I went to one of my favorite coffee shops to spend a few hours applying for jobs. There was a barista there who I thought was cute, but I hadn't really gotten the chance to talk to her. That day, we chatted for a few minutes while I ordered my first coffee, and I learned that not only did we share the same hobby, she was exceptional at it. I knew I had to ask her out.

As I wrapped up for the day a few hours later, I walked past the coffee bar, and even though every bone in my body was screaming at me to take the easy way out and just go home, I stopped and asked her out on a date.

Adrenaline was still surging through my veins when I got home. I started writing a post for the stuttering forum: To tell them that despite my stutter, despite all the turmoil in my life, I went up to a girl, told her I thought she was pretty, and asked her out: If I could do it, so can you.

But I realized that the story from that day wasn't the complete picture. It wouldn't be fair to tell a story of the time I had plucked up the courage to take on a difficult speaking situation, when there were so many other times that I hadn't. The times I had chickened out, or was so nervous that I stuttered terribly. Those experiences were essential; the lessons I gained from those failures were the reason why I was able to succeed that day.

As the paragraphs turned into pages, I realized this wasn't a single post; this wouldn't even fit into a series of posts. *This needs to be a book.*

For two years I wrote solely from my own experience: I explained the experience of stuttering as I knew it and offered advice based on what I had learned. It never occurred to me write about the research on stuttering because I believed the refrain I had heard so often from the stuttering community: "Nobody knows what causes stuttering." "Unfortunately, there just isn't much research about stuttering."

Then, on January 8, 2020, I googled "What causes stuttering?" and a few of the search results were academic studies. The first paper I read was a master's thesis written in the 1980's, a historical overview of supposed causes and "cures" for stuttering, none of which seemed particularly credible. The second paper I read that night was "How The Brain Repairs Stuttering," a 2009 study led by Christian Kell and Katrin Neumann. There was so much information in those fourteen pages that I spent the following three nights just trying to make sense of it.

That paper taught me that intensive speech therapy did in fact work and that, in fact, neuroscientists actually knew quite a bit about how and why stutterers' brains produce stuttered speech. And it reported the L BA 47/12 activation pattern – that the brains of highly-fluent stutterers activate differently than both fluent speakers and other stutterers – which justified my sense that, by that time of my life, I was somehow at my most fluent yet with less struggle.

That study is so rich that I was going to write an entire chapter on it alone, and title it "The Science of Stuttering." That is, until a friend of mine suggested I read the studies cited by Kell and Neumann and then read those studies that cite Kell and Neumann's work.

For the following three months, I spent around twenty hours a week reading research papers. (Harder than I'd ever studied in college.) Anytime my reading brought me across an interesting citation, I'd open another browser tab and read that paper, too. My research started with the neuroscience of stuttering but quickly branched out to genetics, treatment, mental health – anything that would be of value to the community. All told, I believe I read well over two hundred academic papers in their entirety, plus sections of several dozen more.

As fascinating as this research was, I was more blown away by how little of it had made its way into the stuttering community. These studies could do wonders to demystify this peculiar disorder for those affected by it – if only the insights were aggregated in one place and translated from the technical language of academic journals into something a layperson like myself could understand.

This book is my humble attempt to close that chasm. This is the book I would have loved to read in my early twenties, when I was struggling with my stutter, struggling with my life, and felt like there was no way I would ever dig myself out of that hole. While I may be sad that this book did not exist when I most needed it, the hope of helping those who have travelled the same path fills me with joy.

This book, however, is not just a literal translation of the research literature. As an independent author writing for the public, I have significantly more liberty to speculate and speak from personal experience than an academic does when writing for a scientific journal. In this book I have added commentary to research, drawn new connections between studies, and even criticized some research organizations.

I expect there will be some who say that I am unqualified to comment on this research, much less write about it. They have a valid point: I am not trained in neuroscience or any other scientific discipline, nor am I a speech therapist. I do not have a PhD, much less a Masters. My highest academic credential is a liberal arts degree I have never used and an underwhelming 2.45 GPA. (I'm not convinced my grades accurately represent how bad of a student I was.) With a resume like that, how could I dare report on academic research, much less add my own two cents, or even criticize some research?

I preempt these criticisms by pointing out that those who take offense do not have to indict my *resume*; they can come after my *work*. If I have misquoted or misinterpreted studies, it should be easy to point out where I made those errors; rather than say that I must have committed errors because of my background.

Additionally, I hope that this book gives credit and further opportunity to the researchers whose work has enabled it. I find it shocking how some of this work has gone unrecognized and under-appreciated, even within the small world of researchers committed to stuttering. I hope that more attention to stuttering may draw in experts – like Christian Kell and Ritta Salmelin – who can make major contributions to our understanding of stuttering with only one or two publications.

While my aim is to inform the public and make the scholarship in this field more accessible, my greatest apprehension in writing this book was that I would cause harm to a researcher by misrepresenting their work. For that reason, I was incredibly fastidious in reading and re-reading these studies while I wrote about them. I have also done my best to clearly delineate the findings of academic research from my own interpretations, in hopes that my speculations do not contaminate the peer-reviewed research upon which they were founded. If I have made errors in representing a researcher's work, I encourage him or her to reach out to me so that I can issue clarifications online.

Writing this book has been the hardest thing I have ever done. I have never worked this hard or cared so much about anything in my life. Nothing I've experienced before this has given me the same feeling of PURPOSE. The driving force that has kept me on this project for five years has been the hope that I would have a positive, meaningful impact on the lives of others.

I hope reading this book helps you even half as much as writing it has helped me.

March 21, 2023

Words Unspoken

Introduction
Dyslexia, Diabetes, and Dysfluency

Speech is very peculiar. When we speak, we can verbalize thoughts so quickly that we don't even need to picture the words themselves in our mind's eye. This process is so fast, fluent, reliable, and effortless that we rarely think about it. But some people think about their speech all the time.

For people who have a stutter, speech is neither fluent nor effortless; it's an unreliable tool fraught with danger and self-consciousness. For people like myself, there is an underlying unease whenever we speak, because we don't know if our speech systems will cooperate with our minds. Simple tasks like answering an unexpected phone call, being called upon in class, or sharing thoughts in a meeting can become terrifying when you have no idea whether your words will come out smoothly, if at all.

This inability to speak fluently – by itself a small impediment – can easily spiral into a life of despair. Humans need to communicate to fulfill the practical needs in our lives: getting a job, making new connections, even completing mundane tasks, like ordering food at a restaurant. Fear of stuttering can lead to a person avoiding these things, which prevents them from taking care of routine necessities and living a healthy, normal life.

Communication is also a spiritual need. Expressing oneself and connecting with others are fundamental components of human existence; and speech is often the most effective way of doing both. Fear of stuttering can create a vicious cycle where a person feels isolated and craves connection, yet is afraid of interacting with others.

Most people know next-to-nothing about stuttering. This is not so surprising in the case of fluent speakers, because only 1% of adults have a stutter; and even then, the stutter is not always obvious. What's surprising to me is how little most stutterers know about the condition despite living with it their entire lives.

With this in mind, this book has two parallel aims for its two audiences: To explain stuttering to the general public, since that can relieve some of the suffering of stuttering; the same way dyslexia has gone from unknown to common knowledge in my lifetime. Secondly, I want my fellow stutterers to be as informed about their condition as diabetics are about theirs, so everyone can manage their speech in a way that reduces suffering and enables thriving.

Dyslexia: Towards a Cultural Understanding

Dyslexia was formalized as a diagnosis one hundred and fifty years ago, yet as recently as a few decades ago, society knew next-to-nothing about this disorder; this lack of awareness caused greater difficulty and suffering for those with dyslexia. As children, dyslexics often struggled in school and were misdiagnosed with general mental deficits and put in remedial classes. As adults, dyslexics had to worry about being mocked for occasionally struggling to read.

Fortunately, society's awareness about dyslexia has significantly increased in the past thirty years, to the point that the average person is aware of dyslexia at a conceptual level, even if they don't know much about the particulars. Primary school teachers – even those without specialized psychological training – know enough about dyslexia to recognize symptoms in young children and accommodate for them. While it may still be moderately uncomfortable for a person to disclose their dyslexia, the average person is knowledgeable enough that there is no need for further, potentially-embarrassing explanation.

I believe that educating the public about stuttering can lead to similar benefits for stutterers. Much of the pain of stuttering comes from how others sometimes respond to it; be it confusion, well-meaning but less-than-helpful advice, or even outright hostility. If however, a stutterer knows the person they're talking to understands stuttering, it would lead to a more pleasant interaction and better fluency. The average person does not have to make drastic changes to their behavior, let alone feel guilt over their fluent speech; a little understanding and empathy would be enough to have a positive effect on the millions of stutterers around the world.

Diabetes: Better Management for Those Afflicted

Imagine if you were diabetic but unaware of even the basic tenets of the disease. You would experience major swings in energy that defied explanation. Trying to manage it on your own would be baffling; sometimes eating sugary food would cause serious reactions, but at other times, sugary food would rescue you from dangerous episodes. Like diabetes, stuttering can be difficult to understand on one's own, and ineffective management can have a massively negative impact on one's well-being.

Fortunately, if you are diagnosed with diabetes today, all the key information about the disease and how to best manage it can be handed to you in a pamphlet. At that point, it's simply up to you to follow the program. Diabetes will still cause problems and require effortful management, but the potential extreme negative outcomes are unlikely if you are well-informed.

In contrast, many people with a stutter are still baffled by its peculiar nature. I subscribe to an online forum for stuttering, and many basic questions are posted on a regular basis: "Does anybody else stutter badly on their own name?" "Does anybody else stutter more when they're stressed or tired?" "Is stuttering a genetic disorder?"

There is also much confusion within the community about how to manage a stutter. There are many speculative, self-generated theories about the best approach; while much of this advice is on the right track, it is confounded and diluted by the noise of outright-incorrect theories. This can cause further helplessness in the face of stuttering; a person with a stutter can bounce from one approach to the next, each showing promise but ultimately failing, until they lose faith in ever making progress.

Fortunately, research conducted within the last twenty years has illuminated much about stuttering, including: the genetic source of stuttering, the neurological differences between stutterers and fluent speakers, how these differences cause stuttered speech, and the reasons why certain things exacerbate or mitigate dysfluency. Most importantly, these studies offer insight into the treatment programs and approaches that lead to better fluency and quality of life. These findings are backed up by large sample sizes, rigorous methodology, and brain scans. This research suggests – and my personal experience confirms – that one can climb from the worst levels of dysfluency and despair up towards a great level of agency and confidence. Therefore, however dysfluent a stutterer may currently be, there is no reason to believe a life of joy is out of reach.

This book aims to explore the totality of the stuttering experience. The first chapter covers the core facts and unique nature of stuttering, demystifying this peculiar disorder for the general public as well as for stutterers themselves. In the second chapter we'll look at how this speech disorder affects one's interactions and relationships with others. Then we venture into the darkest depths in the third chapter, exploring how – at its worst – a stutter can lead to a life of limitation, despair, and suffering.

Once we've explored the personal side of stuttering and the potential gravity of its effects, we'll catch up on the latest scientific research, starting with childhood development. Chapter four covers the genetic origins and the separate neurological paths that children travel down as their stutter either resolves or persists. Next, we cover what treatments are available for children who have started stuttering and what kind of results a parent can expect.

In chapter six, we'll dive into the neuroscience of speech production; how it works in fluent speakers and exactly where it breaks down in stutterers. Chapter seven explains how speech therapy practices that were developed seventy years ago have recently been shown to counteract these deficits and change stutterers' brains for the better. Chapter eight pulls all of this research together, building a gameplan that any stutterer can use to escape the worst pain of stuttering, improve fluency, and reach stability. Chapter nine lays out the even loftier goal of successful management, where the potential to stutter still exists, but the symbiotic connection between fluency and agency lead to living one's best life. We will cover the personal experience, the neuroscience, and how to get there.

I intersperse these chapters with vignettes from my life: Struggles, successes, and experiences with other stutterers I've met along the way. I hope these stories will help illuminate the inner experience of someone with a stutter.

Chapter One: Fluency and Dysfluency
What Exactly is Stuttering?

Spring 2004

I'm in my senior year English class. The twenty or so of us are sitting in a circle, discussing T.H. White's "The Once and Future King." Our teacher leads a roundtable about the chapters we've read so far, asking which sections we've particularly enjoyed. A few other students raise their hands and answer. I've known most of my classmates for years, and my fluency has been good recently, so I feel comfortable enough to raise my hand, too; I say that I really enjoyed the concept of Merlin experiencing time backwards while everyone else is moving forwards.

All is going fine until our teacher says "Okay everyone, go to page seventy-three. We're going to take turns reading aloud from" I'm in panic mode before she's even finished the sentence.

I may be able to get myself to speak up in class if I'm not having a bad day, but reading aloud almost never goes well. Everyone else will read their sections smoothly and fluently; I'll probably stumble and stutter the whole way through.

My classmates probably know me well enough to realize that I have a stutter, but these exercises are still incredibly unpleasant. Every block I have will hold up the rest of the class. Everyone will be focusing on me, following every word that I should be able to say fluently. Plus, because we're reading from a book, I won't be able to swap difficult words for easier ones if I really get stuck.

Our teacher continues, "We'll start at the third paragraph with Jake, and then we'll go around the room to the left."

I count the number of seats between Jake and me. Then, I count the number of paragraphs starting at Jake's section. I get about halfway down the page before hitting a section of short paragraphs and dialogue, which throws me off even more; I don't know when our teacher will decide that a student has read their quota and can move on. I make my best guess and think I have found what will be my section.

My classmates are reading, but I barely even hear them; I'm hyper-focused on my paragraph. I practice by saying all the words in my head fluently, hoping this silent rehearsal will help me when it's my turn to speak. Deep down, however, I know from experience that this probably won't do anything. I still do it though, because I'm desperate.

In the very last sentence of my paragraph, I see the phrase "When he looked closer..." *Goddammit*, I think.

For my entire life, I've always blocked more on words that start with *cl-* and *gl-*. I can start the motions to pronounce the *cl-* sound, but my mouth freezes when I actually go to say it; my tongue sticks against my top front teeth, my throat closes up, and – rather unpleasantly – I can't push any air out.

I've practiced saying these words at home for hours at a time but it hasn't helped much. Instead, I'm still stressed and anxious about the word, which I know will make me even more likely to block.

The student in front of me nears the end of her paragraph. I'm ready to start speaking the instant she finishes. I don't know why I have this urge – maybe because I associate any bit of silence during my turn with blocking.

I hit the ground reading at one hundred miles an hour. I rush through the paragraph as quickly as possible, hoping that if I go fast enough I won't get stuck. I'm hitting smaller blocks along the way, but I do my best to ignore them and power forward, a speeding truck bouncing all over a backcountry road. The way I'm reading my section, *The Once and Future King* doesn't even sound like a great piece of literature; it's just a blast of words.

I get to the sentence with the *cl-* word and make my first tentative attempt: "Wh-when he looked– When he - looked –"

It's happening, just like I expected. I'm squeezing my diaphragm as hard as I can but no air comes out. The tip of my tongue is hanging up against my front teeth, but I just can't *get it to do the next thing*, to trigger the word "closer" to come out.

I can feel my classmates' discomfort, and it makes me feel guilty; I'm holding everyone up and it's all because of my stupid freaking stutter.

I squeeze and push even harder. I'm leaning forward, as if that will move my speech.

Some invisible trigger finally fires, the catch on mouth releases and the word "closer" shoots out.

I wrap off the last sentence and slam on the brakes. My brain is racing a million miles an hour and my nervous system is still in full fight-or-flight mode, but it's finally over.

I sink down in my chair, feeling exposed and humiliated. I've been reminded that I can't do something so simple that everyone else takes it granted.

I've mostly calmed down by the time the last student, Brad, starts to read. He hates these read-aloud exercises, too, but more out of general apathy towards school. He recites his section in a dull monotone, like he resents even that little bit of effort.

I stare at him and think about the contrast between our experiences: To me, reading aloud in class feels like a life-or-death struggle; Brad is bored out of his mind.

What is Stuttering?

Stuttering is a speech disorder that causes involuntary disruptions – or "blocks" – in one's speech. Stuttering appears all over the world and throughout written history; stuttering-like behavior has even been observed – and induced – in animals. Research estimates that .72% of adults have a stutter.[1] This small number has a skewed gender ratio; for every woman who stutters, there are three men who do.

Blocks are often misinterpreted by those unfamiliar with stuttering. Because fluent speakers have a one-to-one connection between their thoughts and speech, they may wonder if a block is the result of interrupted thoughts, or, conversely, whether a block interrupts one's ability to think. Neither is the case.

Think of blocks the same way as the tremor of Parkinson's disease: the person has a clear intention of what they want to do but the neurological processes that execute this action are not operating correctly.

Blocks come in three varieties: prolongations, repetitions, and hard blocks.

Prolongations are when a syllable is extended longer than the speaker intended, like "I wwwwent to the party." Having a prolongation block feels like you're frozen in time while the rest of the world carries on. It's like that moment that you crest the first hill on a rollercoaster: when you're hanging over the edge, waiting for the release that will send the car hurtling forward.

Repetitions are what most people imagine when they think of stuttering: the speaker repeats a word or syllable multiple times, like "I went to the p-p-p-p-party." Unlike a fluent speaker repeating themselves, during a repetition block the stutterer's mouth will repeat and reset faster than thought, like a machine. Repetitions feel like that moment when you step onto an ice-skating rink and your foot slides out in front of you, and you're helpless to stop it.

Hard blocks are when no sound comes out at all, like "I – – I -w –went to the party." These, in my experience, are the most unpleasant type of blocks. They are like prolongations in that you feel frozen or "stuck," but worse in that no sound, not even air, comes out. The natural instinct is to fight the resistance of the block by pushing harder, but that feels like trying to force repelling magnets together. Sometimes brute force can get you through a block, but more likely, pushing back will only make things works.

I primarily experience hard blocks and, to a lesser degree, prolongations. However, I have met others who almost exclusively have repetitions. Neurological research has yet to conclusively demonstrate this, but I think it is highly like that – while developmental stuttering has a broad, common neurological etiology – minor neurological differences may lead to these variations.

Roughly eight percent of children begin stuttering between the ages of two and four, even if they were fluent when they first begin speaking.[1] However, the vast majority of these children regain fluency in the months or years that follow and never stutter again. When a stutter persists into adolescence, it almost always becomes a lifelong affliction.

While this book is about *developmental* stuttering there are other, less-common etiologies. *Neurogenic* stuttering is caused by damage to the brain through a stroke or other physical trauma. While stress tends to exacerbate a developmental stutter, *psychogenic* stuttering is itself caused by extreme emotional distress, and can be resolved through therapeutic counseling.

Developmental stuttering, on the other hand, has a genetic source and leads to a particular neurological outcome. Contrary to older theories, developmental stuttering is not caused by traumatic events in childhood, a child's personality, or other environmental factors.

Blocks occur unpredictably and are beyond a stutterer's control; while it is possible to manage fluency, no amount of intention or effort can *guarantee* fluency on any given word a stutterer says. Furthermore, for adult stutterers, this proclivity to block will never go away entirely; a stutterer is liable to block on any word they will ever say, for the rest of their lives.

Quirks of Stuttering

A stutter's fluency can vary dramatically from situation to situation and over the course of one's life. Generally speaking, fluency improves when one is calm, confident, and in control. Fluency also tends to increase with age and maturity as one becomes more experienced in managing fluency and themselves. There can also be good days and bad days that defy explanation.

In addition to these larger ebbs and flows, there are also quirks of language that increase or decrease fluency in the moment. Stutterers are more likely to block on the first syllable of a word and on the first word in a sentence. Additionally, having a history of blocking on a particular word can cause a stutterer to develop anxiety over that particular word, increasing the stress and tension in a self-perpetuating cycle of stress, anxiety, and dysfluency.

Stutterers also have an unusual proclivity to block on their own names. Perhaps it comes from the pressure of being put on the spot by a question that should be quick and easy to answer.

There are also "nemesis phonemes†," those on which a particular speaker is most likely to block. I struggle most on words that start with *cl-* or *gl-* but I know some stutterers who block more often on words starting with *s-* or *p-*.

For some reason, stutterers are more likely to block when asked to repeat themselves, even if they were perfectly fluent the first time. I've experienced this myself; when someone asks me to repeat myself, it suddenly feels like the ground I'm standing on has become unsteady.

For neurological reasons that we will explore later, stutterers are also more likely to block on syntactically-complex words. *Syntactic complexity* refers to how complicated the sounds are in a particular word or syllable – rather than the complexity of thought or ideas, which is "semantic complexity." The phrases "elevated syntactic

---

† A *phoneme* is the basic unit of sound in a language. For example, the word "twist" is only one syllable, but contains five phonemes: t/w/i/s/t.

complexity" and "a lot of big words" mean the same thing, but the former is more syntactically complex than the latter.

It's an interesting quirk of stuttering that one may become obstinately stuck on a particular word but fluently glide through another, even if those two words mean the same thing. This is why stutterers will often use "word substitution" to preemptively avoid a block. Because I struggle with *cl-* sounds, I frequently substituted the word "course" for "class" during my school years. The word "classroom" does not have an obvious synonym, but if I needed to get around it. I might've said something clumsy like "the room where it's at."

I met an older gentleman at a stuttering support group who, whenever he introduced himself, emphasized that his name was *Eugene* Johnson. He explained that even though he always preferred the name "Eugene," he went by "Gene" for decades because he was afraid of stuttering over his own name. I've even heard more than one story of stutterers lying about their own name to avoid dysfluency.

Another strategy sometimes used to avoid a block is "feigned ignorance." By pretending to not remember the word for something, the stutterer can wait for someone else to interject and say that word for them.

Alternatively, in order to build momentum against an anticipated block, sometimes stutterers will add "bridge words" into their speech. This may mean adding in "um's," "uh's," or even whole words. The most recognizable example comes from the actor Samuel L. Jackson, who is notorious for how often he says the word "m--------er" in his film roles. Jackson, who has a stutter, once explained that he inserted more than a few of these "m--------er's" into his lines to get past a block.

There are also other quirks of speech that can induce perfect fluency. Stutterers will become perfectly fluent when singing, whispering, putting on an accent, or speaking in time to a metronome. The quirk about being fluent while singing adds great irony to the song "My Generation" by The Who. The song's lyrics famously imitate a stutter: "Talking bout my ge-ge-generation..." A stutterer may talk like that, but because singing induces perfect fluency, they would never *sing* like that.

Another fluency-inducing mechanism is an audio distortion called "delayed auditory feedback" (DAF) wherein a person wears headphones that play back their own speech with a small delay. Hearing one's own speech with a tiny delay of sixty milliseconds is enough to make stutterers perfectly fluent. This is the mechanism behind the SpeechEasy, an in-ear device for stutterers that can lead to significantly-improved fluency, though the effect wears off with time.

I once saw unintentional DAF in action during a presentation at a conference. The presenter was severely dysfluent, but when he spoke directly into the microphone, the playback from the speakers was loud enough to reach him on stage; the minor delay that came from the sound traveling from the audio system to him inadvertently created a DAF effect. However, whenever he turned his head away from the microphone to gesture at his slides, the volume from the speakers went down, and since he was no longer hearing his speech on a slight delay, his fluency regressed.

Stuttering Beyond Speech

At its core, stuttering is not a disorder peculiar to speech, but one that encompasses the motor expression of language more generally; those who stutter exhibit blocks in other modalities in surprising ways.

I experience minor blocks while writing and have heard similar reports from other stutterers. When this happens, my hand will inexplicably hang for a second at the beginning of a curve, like a prolongation, then carry on at a normal pace once it passes that stroke. Or, like a hard block, my pen sometimes freezes at the very beginning of a letter. Like with syntactically-complex speech, these written blocks happen most often for me on technically-complex characters like "m," "S," and "3."

Another example of manual stuttering comes from a group of people who may rarely speak: the deaf and hard of hearing. These deaf "stutterers" exhibit blocks while signing in American Sign Language. In his college honor's thesis, Geoff Whitebread listed eight different expressions of blocks in the hearing-impaired, many of which are very similar to spoken blocks. Signers would have difficulty initiating signs, or would repeat smaller parts of a sign, or would hold one motion in a sign longer than normal.[2] Professor Jody Cripps noted that the 3:1 male-female ratio of stuttering signers matched that of stuttering speakers. Stuttering signers were also more likely to block while finger-spelling, which is reasonably analogous to syntactic complexity in speech.[3]

Researcher Greg Snyder wrote about his experience as a stutterer who communicates via "SimCom" – speaking and signing at the same time. When he paid closer attention to his hands while his speech blocked, he noticed that his signing stopped too, as if his hands were "waiting" for his speech before continuing. After noticing this, he trained his hands to continue signing even while he was stuck on a verbal block. He could maintain these two separate streams of language until his hands were an entire phrase ahead of his speech, at which point he would need to "reset" and bring his hands back to where his speech was.[4]

An even more strange apparition of stuttering has been observed in music. One flutist reported difficulty in playing the first note of songs, like how stutterers are most likely to block on the first word of a sentence. Snyder wrote about a man who reported similar disruptions while playing the trumpet: "As one who stuttered... it feels *exactly* the same. In fact, it *was* stuttering." This trumpet player also struggled with the complex techniques of double- and triple-tonguing, going so far as to avoid songs with those techniques the way stutterers avoid troublesome words.[4]

A quick sidebar on terminology: Some people in the community prefer the term "person who stutters" over "stutterer" because the former is ostensibly gentler, and the latter could imply that a person is defined by their stutter. I believe the most accurate term would be "person *who has* a stutter" because the stutter is something external that happens to you, whereas "person who stutters" inaccurately suggests that the stutter is something a person *does*, like a "person who golfs."

In this book, I primarily use the term "stutterer" because it's short and simple, but you can read it to mean "person who has a stutter". While the term "dysfluent" isn't used much at the moment, I think it would be a useful term because of its similarity to the way we say someone is "dyslexic."

If you are a fluent speaker and you're referring to someone who has a stutter, any term you use is fine by me. I don't speak for everyone, but I won't be offended by your word choice as long as you're not deliberately trying to insult me.

And for what it's worth, I think the debate over terminology is a bit frivolous; I believe that the reality of having a stutter is heavier than whatever term you use to describe it, and soft language can only do so much to relieve that burden.

More Than Just Speech

Having a stutter is more than just a difference in the way someone speaks. Human beings are social creatures, and speech is (usually) the fastest and easiest way to communicate; a stutter affects how you experience all social interactions. Even if the other person doesn't know that you have a stutter, *you* know that you may block, and *you* have to navigate your speech around dysfluency. After all, you never know how someone will respond to your stutter. While blocking may be viscerally unpleasant, the way others react to your dysfluency is probably the most painful part of having a stutter.

What about one's relationship to other stutterers? On one hand, fellow stutterers are likely to have shared similar experiences, and you could reach a deep level of connection of empathy and understanding.

However, a stutter is often a very sensitive subject, especially when someone feels powerless over their own speech.

Let's look at the social world through the eyes of someone who has a stutter.

Chapter Two: Stuttering in the Social World
Aversion, Discomfort, and Support

Spring 2017

I was visiting an old Coast Guard buddy of mine and looking for activities we could do together. I had always thought my friend would like Brazilian jiu-jitsu, considering how much he loved the wrestling matches that sometimes broke out in the living quarters of the ship we had been stationed on together.

Before my trip, I found a jiu-jitsu gym five minutes from his house that looked perfect. The owner of the gym, "Jack," had earned his black belt under a respected teacher, so I trusted his credentials. On top of that, Jack was a retired Special Forces operator who had done multiple tours in Afghanistan and Iraq, then went back to the Middle East with the CIA. On top of that, he surfed – so not only was he a qualified jiu-jitsu instructor, he seemed pretty badass.

I was really excited to call Jack and ask whether my friend and I – amateurs – could drop in on his Saturday morning class. My excitement wasn't just about going to the class: Seven years earlier I had called a jiu-jitsu gym near my hometown to ask about signing up. At the time, my dysfluency was pretty bad, and my fear of phone calls only made it worse. I was so embarrassed by how badly I stuttered that I almost didn't even show up for my first class.

Since that call, my fluency and confidence had gotten much better; while calling a stranger on the phone was still difficult, I could handle it. I looked forward to calling Jack because I saw it as a serendipitous opportunity to overwrite that earlier, disastrous call.

So I was surprised and a little disappointed when I couldn't find a phone number listed anywhere on the gym's website. I settled for sending an emailing instead, and Jack replied that he would be happy to have us.

The morning of the class my friend and I checked in. Jack was telling us what to expect from the class when I noticed a slight halt in his speech. I paid closer attention to the way he talked, and after another slightly unnatural bump, I was positive: *Jack had a stutter, too.*

But I didn't tell Jack about my stutter, much less say anything about his. I almost never out myself when I think I've met another stutterer. I didn't know how Jack would respond to the topic, and I was still a bit intimidated by his resume.

Jack was a great instructor and his class was a lot of fun. We drilled techniques and sparred with members of the gym; my friend absolutely loved it.

Near the end of the class, Jack was demonstrating the finer points of a particular technique, when he said "Now a trick used a lot by uh... by uh... ah, what's his name..." He shook his head and snapped his fingers like the name was on the tip of his tongue. "The Brazilian guy who won at Worlds last year... the heavyweight from Sao Paulo..."

I'm not a mind reader, but I strongly suspected Jack was just feigning ignorance, an avoidance technique I was all too familiar with.

A student said "You mean *Buchecha*?"

"Oh yeah, that's his name!" Jack said, and continued on with his explanation.

This episode floored me. Jack had volunteered to face death in combat zones, had reached the pinnacle of a grueling sport, and had been in an elite branch of the military – yet in his own gym, surrounded by people who knew him very well, even *he* used avoidance techniques.

It wasn't until a few days later, as I drove home, that I was struck by another realization: Maybe Jack didn't list a phone number on his website because he didn't want unexpected calls from strangers.

Having a stutter doesn't just affect the way you feel when you speak; it affects how others feel when you speak, too. Others may notice that something is "off" about stutterers' speech, even if they can't put a finger on the reason, and will feel uncomfortable around dysfluency. And with a lifetime's experience of speaking to others, stutterers easily pick up on the discomfort of the people they interact with. For this reason, stuttering doesn't just affect speech: It affects interpersonal relationships as a whole.

Unexpected and Unfamiliar

Multiple studies have found that fluent speakers have a different reaction to the speech of stutterers than fluent speakers. This was true for students, parents, speech–language clinicians, special educators, people who stutter, vocational rehabilitation counsellors, teachers, and professors.[5]

A more-recent pair of studies led by Vijaya Guntupalli examined how fluent speakers reacted to someone with a stutter. In the studies, fluent speakers watched one-minute videos of people speaking; the participants were not told in advance that half of the speakers had a severe stutter. In the first study, participants rated how the videos made them feel on an emotional spectrum, such as nervous versus calm or comfortable versus uncomfortable. Compared to the videos of the fluent speakers, participants reported the stutterers' video made them feel more unhappy, nervous, uncomfortable, sad, tense, unpleasant, avoiding, embarrassed, and annoyed by the stutterers' videos.[6]

While the results of the first study were based on self-reported emotions, the second focused on measurable physical outcomes. In that study, Guntupalli found that fluent speakers had autonomic responses while watching videos of stutterers speaking. They showed increased electrical conductance on their skin, which is associated with a stress response. Additionally, their heart rate slowed down, which he interpreted as akin to a fear response.[7]

To my mind, natural, uncoached reactions like confusion or distaste are totally understandable responses to a stutter. A stutterer who is blocking is clearly trying to speak – something nearly every other person can do effortlessly – but that is disrupted by some invisible, intangible force. When a person doesn't know that these blocks come from a speech disorder, they may wonder if they are part of a larger neurological or mental health issue. After all, only one in a hundred adults have a stutter – and even then it is not always apparent – so the average person isn't likely to have much experience or knowledge surrounding stuttering.

For fluent speakers, eye contact is also an expected part of conversation; if someone doesn't make eye contact, the behavior is perceived as nervousness or even dishonesty. However, many stutterers, myself included, often avoid eye contact while speaking. Maintaining eye contact during a block can be very unpleasant; in a way, it draws the listener into the experience of your block and exposes you to the often-unpleasant reaction on their face. I've also found the intensity of eye contact is liable to trip up my fluency.

Some things stutterers do in an attempt to mitigate dysfluency can further exacerbate the discomfort of an interaction. *Secondary behaviors* are tic-like actions that aim to improve fluency by bridging into speech with some kind of motion, or a way to release physical energy when one's speech articulators are blocked. They can be as mild as furrowing one's brow or leaning slightly forward; they can also be as extreme as flapping one's hands or making non-speech sounds. These crutch-like habits – however effective they may feel – do not actually improve fluency but may increase the listener's discomfort.

While it is unpleasant when someone gets noticeably uncomfortable with my speech, I try not to take it personally. These reactions are not malicious or mean-spirited; they come from interpreting stuttering through the lens of what someone knows. I have been guilty of judging others' speech or behavior through the lens of normalcy, only to later discover an underlying cause like Tourette's or even a stutter. It's not surprising that fluent speakers may find stuttering surprising or uncomfortable – stutterers themselves don't necessarily have a comfortable relationship to seeing someone else stutter either.

A Surprising Distance Between Stutterers

It's strange that stutterers have a commonality that has a huge impact on our lives, and we make up such a small part of the population that it's quite rare to meet one another, yet – in my experience – we may never talk about it.

One of my closest friends in college had a stutter. We spent hundreds of hours together and shared some deeply personal matters with each other, but neither of us ever acknowledged each other's blocks or so much as said the word "stutter." My first boss in the Coast Guard had a stutter, too. We worked together for almost a year, spending half of that time at sea – an environment where interpersonal barriers break down, and others see past your surface-level self-projection – but we never spoke about stuttering.

I think we stutterers may avoid bringing it up with each other because if you have a stutter, you know what a painful, personal subject it can be. Many stutterers – and I have felt this way in the past – would rather forget about it entirely.

I didn't want to think about my stutter when I was younger, much less talk to another person about it. Unpleasant speaking experiences were still a regular occurrence and could happen at any time, so it was uncomfortable for me to see someone else block or struggle with their fluency. If I saw stuttering in a movie, or met someone who had a stutter, I would actively distance myself from it.

I'm sure there are stutterers who are much more likely to broach the subject with new acquaintances; more power to them. For me, however, it would still seem too forward to draw attention to another person's stutter, even if it was only to put them at ease. This may be overly-tentative of me, but in my defense, I've never had another stutterer bring it up with me, either.

That said, there is at least one environment where stuttering is openly discussed: stuttering support groups.

Stuttering Support Groups

I went to my first stuttering support group at the age of thirty-four. I hadn't gone before then because I never really considered the stutter to be a major part of my identity; it was just an obstacle to navigate while I did other things. I didn't think the meeting would affect me on a personal or emotional level because I felt at peace with my stutter; the worst times were in the past and I knew how to manage it going forward. By that time, I was already writing this book; I had been thinking about stuttering everyday for two years and reliving some of my most painful experiences while I wrote about them, so I was expecting the experience to be one of sympathetic but detached observation.

But I was wrong. Hearing a story of suffering or hardship from another person – especially when I had experienced the same thing – was more poignant than I had expected; I found myself fighting back tears several times. I wasn't sorry for the experiences I had gone through, but seeing someone else suffer made me sympathetic towards others in a way that I rarely am with myself. You get accustomed to brushing off the bumps and bruises that come with having a stutter; but when you spend time talking and listening to others, you feel the full weight of what you've all been dealing with.

In the first meetup I went to, a woman in her thirties broke down crying in the middle of a roundtable discussion simply because she had never met another person who stuttered, and now she was surrounded by them. She wasn't alone in this feeling: A friend of mine went to a three-day stuttering conference, and was so emotionally overwhelmed by the sense of community that he broke down sobbing during his flight home.

A stuttering support group is such a novel environment for someone who has spent their entire life in a fluent world. It can be freeing to speak without worrying about your stutter, or whether someone will react unfavorably to it. And because stuttering has no correlation with personal traits or background, these support groups attract people with all kinds of different personalities, careers, and hobbies who are nonetheless connected at a deep level by their shared experience.

Uncharitable Responses

While stuttering groups provide community, everyday experiences can be much more isolating. Some responses are deliberately intended to cause hurt, while others are not really meant to cause offense but may still be unpleasant.

The phrase "*Did I stutter?!*" is an American colloquialism that means something like "Do I need to repeat myself?!" I was once out dancing with friends when the DJ interrupted the music to yell that at some hooligan in the crowd. It didn't feel good to be reminded of my stutter while I was out having fun with my friends, but at the same time, it's not like that phrase is meant to insult or demean stutterers. Maybe we could replace that phrase with something better, but I don't think it makes people think less of stutterers, so I'm not going to invest time or effort to remove it from the public lexicon. I have more control over my own reactions than what other people say.

In *South Park*, one of my favorite tv shows, there is a character named Jimmy who has a stutter, and it's often used for comedic effect.† When Jimmy was first introduced to the show, it made me a little upset that the show's

---

† In the *South Park* video game *The Stick of Truth*, right before the start of a climactic battle Jimmy delivers the line "Step forward now and fulfill your destiny!" but he blocks on the end of "destiny." He repeats the full phrase, but again blocks on the last word and starts the whole phrase over. This cycle goes on for such an uncomfortably long time that the game actually gives the player the option to skip to the end of the scene. I think the bit is actually quite clever; and judging by the YouTube comments, I'm not the only stutterer who finds it funny.

creators were purposefully placing the character in situations where his stutter was the butt of the joke. But I got used to it after a few episodes; I had to remind myself that the whole point of *South Park*'s sense of humor – which, admittedly, is not for everyone – is that *everyone* is fair game. It wouldn't be fair for me to laugh when they joke that redheads don't have souls but then be upset when stuttering is the target du jour.

Unfortunately, sometimes others will deliberately target you because of your stutter. Having a stutter makes you a prime target for bullying, as the speech impediment is a clear difference that a bully can use to mark someone as different, weird, or "less-than." Additionally, having a stutter makes it harder for a person to verbally defend themselves. In a study of adolescents, the husband-and-wife team of Gordon and Ingrid Blood found that while only 11% of fluent adolescents were at risk of experiencing bullying behavior, 43% of stuttering adolescents were. They also screened participants for poor communicative ability, a factor that correlated with increased risk of bullying victimization. While only 11% of the fluent children rated themselves as having poor communicative ability, 57% of the stuttering children reported they did.[8]

I have even heard people mock stuttering when speaking to me, not knowing that I have a stutter. I was once talking to a Coastie from another unit, and we were trying to see if we knew anyone in common. When I mentioned my previous boss – the one who had a stutter – this guy said "Oh, that stuttering idiot?"

I'm not absolving all bad behavior, but I think the worst reactions are bad attempts to release the subconscious tension and discomfort that comes from listening to a dysfluent person speak. For whatever reason, humans tend to notice when a person speaks abnormally. We falsely attribute a speech difference – be it stuttering, a lisp, a foreign accent – as a conscious failure of that person to speak properly, even when on a rational level, we know it's beyond the speaker's control. The Monty Python movie *The Life of Brian* uses a variety of these speech differences – stuttering, lisping, pronouncing *r*'s and *l*'s like *w*'s – as comedic fodder. We find it ironic that Mike Tyson has a lisp because we attribute a lisp to a soft, almost weak disposition. Even today, when we want to imply a person is not very smart, we usually lower our voice and dull our enunciation.

Specifically for stuttering, there is an inescapable tension when someone blocks and it's obvious what they mean to say afterwards. If we know exactly what is coming, but we have to wait for it to arrive, that unpredictability can feel a little irritating or tiring; it demands patience. I've felt that tension – a subconscious urge to say "spit it out!" – even though I am intimately familiar with the unpleasantness of blocking.

While educating the public will improve the way society responds to stuttering, I think we should also set reasonable expectations. It's unrealistic to expect that every single person will always respond kindly to stuttering; there will always be people who react with impatience, rudeness, or outright hostility. We can't control how others act, but we can affect how we feel, and we can choose how we respond.

That said, there are many kind and empathetic fluent speakers who would be happy to do what they can to accommodate stuttering and make our lives easier.

Advice For Fluent Speakers

Every person with a stutter is an individual with their own preferences. Some are happy to talk about it if asked respectfully; others are not. For fluent speakers who are looking to respond to stuttering in a helpful way, I would encourage kindness and curiosity, but also respect for stutterers who do not want attention drawn to their speech.

If you notice someone has a stutter but seems unbothered by however fluent they are, I generally wouldn't recommend bringing attention to it. In such cases, I think the best thing you can do is treat them like you would any other person, albeit with a bit of extra patience for their speech.

If you're talking with someone who seems to be struggling on a personal level – rather than just blocking – I think it is okay to say something like "I'm sorry to interrupt, and I don't mean to be presumptuous, but I noticed you might have a stutter. I just want to offer that I understand a little about stuttering, and you don't have to worry about being misjudged. I'm here."

A small gesture like that could make a stutterer's life a lot easier.

Some fluent speakers might feel like they "don't have the right" to say that they understand stuttering. I've even heard a long-tenured and well-respected speech pathologist say, with an air of semi-guilt, "I could never *truly* understand what it's like to live with a stutter." As a stutterer, I don't agree with that sentiment. A fluent speaker may never directly experience the anxiety of wondering whether or not their words will come out, but anxiety itself is pretty universal. Maybe a fluent speaker will never feel the unique physical sensations of blocking, but empathy and imagination can get you pretty close.

It is true that stuttering is a unique phenomenon with its own particular downstream effects, but the biggest hurdle to understanding what it's like to have a stutter is simply knowing the basic nature of stuttering. (And, to my mind, by reading this far into the book, you've made it.)

Even though every person has a wildly different life experience, our shared humanity trumps these minor differences. After all, people are people.

We stutterers want and need those feelings of connection and empathy with the people around us; without them, a stutter can lead to a very dark place.

Chapter Three: Suffering
Withdrawal, Despair, and Hopelessness

January 2018

There is a particular kind of post that frequently appears in a stuttering forum I subscribe to. These posts start with the user venting about a recent stuttering experience that was especially painful. Maybe they stuttered really badly during a presentation, or someone laughed at the way they talk, or an authority figure chastised them for not being a better speaker. But then, the poster quickly moves from describing this one incident into admitting that it feels like their stutter is constricting their entire life. These posts are equal parts solicitation for advice and cry for help. I've seen dozens of discussion threads like this – they appear about once a week – but one from January 2018 was so poignant that it has stayed with me ever since.

This particular poster, a young man who had recently graduated high school, began by venting about his inability to land a job. He had already been on a handful of interviews, but they were all disasters. He was always nervous about how the interviewers would respond to his stutter, and the stress caused his stutter to flare up even worse than usual. Dysfluency prevented him from answering questions the way he wanted to, and his interviewers – who didn't seem to know much about stuttering – simply thought he was nervous or incompetent.

After being passed over for jobs he wanted, he swallowed his pride and applied for any job he could get. Even when he was overqualified, his dysfluency and lack of confidence turned off interviewers. By the time he wrote this post, he had just about given up on job-hunting altogether and resigned himself to the fact that he couldn't afford to move out of his parents' house.

His social life wasn't doing much better. As a recent high school graduate who didn't go to college, he was no longer surrounded by friends and peers. The isolation was unpleasant and he desperately wanted to be more social, but he was terrified of striking up conversations with strangers or going out to gatherings by himself. So he spent most of his time at home, living like a shut-in. To make matters worse, he wasn't even safe there; his family frequently mocked his stutter.

This young man's nascent adult life had failed to launch and he was clearly suffering. He should have been out exploring the new possibilities of life as an independent adult or making friends in the next stage of his life. Instead, he had no friends, no self-confidence, and nothing to do with his time. He felt like his stutter was preventing him from making any kind of progress towards the life he wanted. He knew that his situation was dire, and he desperately wanted to get a grip on his speech, but nothing he tried ever seemed to work.

At the close of his post, he wrote that thoughts about the future filled him with dread. He was already behind his peers, and the gap was expanding, not closing. He didn't see how he was going to dig himself out of this hole. The worst case scenarios seemed very probable to him. Was he going to experience nothing but this miserable, limited existence for the next sixty years? What if his life got even smaller?

Feeling like he had no other options, he closed by writing something I'll never forget: "If I believed in reincarnation, I would just kill myself and hope to be reborn as someone without a stutter."

Having a stutter isn't just the experience of interrupted speech; it's the wear and tear of your body not cooperating with your mind, the unpleasant social reactions to your speech, and the seeming hopelessness of ever getting a grip on fluency.

These problems can spiral into the bottomless suffering the young man above experienced. In fact, I would bet that most stutterers have experienced a period of deep despair and hopelessness at least once in their lives. Research on the mental health of stutterers supports this bleak picture.

Social anxiety is clinically defined[9] as "Persistent, intense fear or anxiety about specific social situations because you believe you may be judged, embarrassed or humiliated. Avoidance of anxiety-producing social situations or enduring them with intense fear or anxiety. *Excessive anxiety that's out of proportion to the situation.*" (Emphasis mine.) That description fits how many stutterers experience the social world: Living with a constant fear of being embarrassed by one's dysfluency, or being humiliated by others with no ability to verbally defend oneself.

Multiple studies have compared stutterers' rates of social anxiety to those of fluent speakers. Figures vary, but at any given moment, about 4% of the general population meets the criteria for a social anxiety diagnosis. That same figure for stutterers is 40%, *ten times* the rate of fluent speakers.[10] One study found that stutterers had substantially-elevated feelings of inadequacy and social inferiority.[11]

A 2011 study led by Yvonne Tran assessed the mood symptoms of stutterers and fluent speakers, and compared them against psychiatric outpatients – that is, people regularly going to therapy for a mood disorder like depression, anxiety, or obsessive-compulsive disorder. Stutterers and fluent speakers were not much different when it came to levels of distress that would require intervention; 30% of fluent speakers had distress scores typical of psychiatric outpatients, compared to 40% of stutterers. Differences became more stark when the researchers calculated which participants were within two standard deviations of the outpatients, meaning they may not need immediate intervention, but they were still struggling. Only 11% of fluent speakers were within this range, compared to a whopping 55% of stutterers. That implies that even if these stutterers weren't at their breaking point, they were still experiencing significantly more duress than the average fluent speaker.[11]

In a 2009 study, Lisa Iverach gave a mental health assessment to stutterers who were on a waitlist for speech therapy. Compared to the general population, this group had six-to-seven times the usual rate of any mental health diagnosis, six times the rate of panic disorders, and four times the rate of generalized anxiety disorder over the previous twelve months.[12]

In another 2009 study, Daniel Craig used questionnaires to compare the impact of stuttering on one's life to that of serious medical conditions. He found that stuttering correlated with decreases in mental health, vitality, and social and emotional functioning. The negative effects on mental health were on par with those that result from quadriplegia or from suffering a traumatic brain injury. The effects on vitality and social-emotional function were similar to those found in people with diabetes and coronary heart disease.[13]

What could explain these drastic effects on mental health? What does this suffering look like at the personal level? For that, we can look to direct quotes from two studies – one by Joseph Corcoran & Moira Stewart, and the other led by Laura Plexico – that included long, open-ended interviews with stutterers about their experience living with dysfluency.[14,15] As Corcoran and Stewart wrote, "To read the participants' accounts of their experience of stuttering is to be confronted by their profound suffering, as evidenced by their reports of nightmares, humiliation, dread, isolation, and thoughts of suicide."

The Burden of Stuttered Speech

These elevated rates of social anxiety make sense when you consider what it's like to go out into the world with a stutter. I don't necessarily feel shame or blame myself when I block, but there's almost always at least a little bit of irritation. Blocks are an unforeseen delay that require extra effort on something trivial. And it's the reappearance of a problem, a sudden reminder that I have a little more weight on my shoulders. Not only does a block stop me from moving forward; it also lays an unexpected problem in my path. And a block is no simple problem to solve.

Each block is unique; working through a block requires feeling out that particular situation – and that demands patience, attention, and effort. This is complicated by the fact that it's impossible to know *when* you will get to the other side.

Having a stutter means facing not just the physical or emotional unpleasantness of blocking; it also means dealing with the *threat* of blocking. The unpredictable nature of blocks can produce a constant state of tension and fear, as one study participant related:

"So much of it is internal. Before the physical matters begin to manifest, you go through all this emotional turmoil.

It's: 'Can I? Can't I? Can I? Can't I?' ... [With] stuttering, you don't know what's going to happen, how it's going to work out this time. People just don't realize."

The constant danger of being called to speak when you go out into the world makes leaving the house feel like stepping into a gladiatorial arena. Even when running an errand that doesn't require speaking to anyone, a stranger may put you on the spot by suddenly approaching you to ask for directions. Phone calls, which are especially difficult for stutterers, have become an ever-present threat now that we all carry phones in our pockets. As one participant related, "I would get totally freaked out by the phone ringing. Like my whole body would go into shock when the phone rang because I knew that I would have to answer it."

Interestingly, Plexico's interviewees weren't just concerned about the distress their stutter caused them; they felt that it was their responsibility to not let their stutter upset the listener, either. As one participant said, "I just don't want to make somebody feel uncomfortable. In essence, I'm okay with it. I know I'm stuttering. I know it's bad. I know there's an awkward silence or an awkward pause. But I don't want you to feel bad."

Another interviewee felt the need to present as more fluent even in an environment where her well-being was the stated priority: "When I was in [speech] therapy in junior high I would substitute and I would not stutter and [my speech therapist] would think that I was making progress, but I was hiding it the whole time. I don't know why I would hide it from the speech pathologist, but I was ashamed of it, so any chance I could dodge a block I took it. So she thought I was making so much progress."

When you consider that the average person doesn't know much about stuttering – and doesn't have the ability to recognize a block for what it is – it makes sense that some stutterers worry about the listener's reaction. One interviewee described the feelings of anxiety that her speech impediment caused: "I thought [listeners] would look down on me because I stuttered... Any four-year-old child can speak fluently. I wasn't accepted as a mature person."

Unsurprisingly, the potential for an interaction to turn sour led participants to spend a significant amount of effort monitoring a listener's body language, checking whether the listener had picked up on the stutter or was becoming annoyed by the speaker's dysfluency.

These feelings gets worse when someone responds to the stutter with outright mockery or hostility. The day I reported to my first Coast Guard unit, I hung out with my new co-workers over drinks. One of them started giggling, and then whispered to the person next to him while gesturing my way. I couldn't tell what they were laughing about, but it already made me uncomfortable. The next time I spoke I noticed they were watching me extra closely; when I had a minor block the first co-worker leaned over to the other and said "See? See?"

For the rest of the night, anytime I spoke they would lean in and stare at my mouth. I didn't want to get into a confrontation with my co-workers on my first day, but I was also worried that I would stutter badly if I tried to stand up for myself, which would only make the situation worse. In the end, I did nothing except bite my tongue and stew.

Given the constant threat that comes with speaking, sometimes one needs relief from the danger, the tension, the pain and the lack of control. As one study participant said, "You know you're always worried about it, obviously you're stuttering like mad... Yeah so it's just both mentally and physically exhausting."

When a person feels like there is no way to mitigate their dysfluency, there is one easy way out: withdrawal and avoidance.

Withdrawal and Avoidance

When a stressor becomes more than a person can tolerate, they can gain control and relief by running away from the problem. For all nine of Plexico's interviewees, withdrawal and avoidance "were perceived as necessary for providing momentary relief from stuttering, preventing emotional suffering, achieving distance from the problem, and for obtaining control over a perceivably uncontrollable situation."

For stutterers, this can mean avoiding speech or escaping oneself during speech. Interviewees in the studies did this with "avoidance, repression, self-distraction, and substance abuse. These methods provided the participants distance from the problem and momentary relief."

Some stutterers turn to drugs or alcohol after they find themselves being more fluent or less self-conscious when inebriated, as one interviewee described: "I would feel really discouraged and it would increase the amount that I would drink. When I was eighteen I found out that alcohol miraculously made me more fluent and I latched onto it. Alcohol was both my liquid courage and liquid fluency."

Drugs and alcohol may provide temporary benefits, but like many avenues of avoidance and withdrawal, they come with longer-term penalties. Habitual avoidance can lead to developing an unhealthy dependence on the only thing that seems to work, even when you know the crutch is a double-edged sword. The interviewee above continued:

"I don't drink before every situation because that's just not good. ... I've discovered that sometimes certain pills help me, which has made me take pain killers. I've gone to the extent of taking them at work and that's not good."

These coping mechanisms hurt, as this interviewee said, because you know that you are relying on unhealthy crutches, rather than developing strength. It's easy to feel stuck between a rock and a hard place: If you cannot solve the problem of the stutter, the only alternative is to rely on these crutches. Knowing that you need to rely on these crutches hurts a person at the deep level of self-confidence, sense of agency, and self-expression; because you know these are the easy way out.

The more one relies on these crutches, the more they become both more harmful and more addictive. As Plexico wrote, "The natural coping pattern of avoidance and escape became a strategy to be relied upon and soon became habituated and difficult to relinquish." I can attest from my own experience that avoidance and withdrawal can spiral into a vicious cycle.

This phenomenon leads to what I call the "momentum meter" of stuttering. If you run away from a challenge – and you continue to run away – your baseline fluency starts to feel worse, and the temptation to withdraw becomes harder to avoid. If you fall into the habit of avoiding speech, this momentum can take you so low that it can feel nigh-impossible to turn the ship around.

Once this vicious cycle begins, it is hard to stop. When you are trapped by negative momentum, you avoid speech because you are afraid of stuttering, but your inability to motivate yourself to speak – your failure to even *try* to speak – makes you further afraid of dysfluency. This can lead to a limited life, one filled with anxiety at the simple thought of speaking. And once you're suffering like this, it's hard to imagine you'll ever get out.

Hopelessness and Despair

As one participant said, "When you stutter, you feel that you have no [control over] your life. You kind of just flop around doing hopefully the easiest thing that comes along and hopefully you'll get by without too much pain."

Faced with the negative impact of withdrawal and avoidance, many stutterers try to improve their fluency. This, sometimes, is easier said than done. A stutterer may try to control their speech articulators more closely, for example, which could lead to improved fluency in the beginning, but then inevitably regress to baseline, or worse. When one strategy fails, there is often another to take its place; perhaps an online tip for self-optimization – a new diet, routine or "lifehack" – may be the next promising approach; but it, too, may offer short-term improvements but no lasting change.

When a person expends significant effort only to fail over and over again, this may result in *learned helplessness*. Corcoran and Stewart summarized a study on the subject, writing "The primary characteristic of learned helplessness was [participants] learning that outcomes were independent of their responding. Nothing [they] did made a difference in the outcomes."

This makes despair deeper: You have a problem now, it will continue to be a problem, and nothing you do seems to make it better. This leads to a painful hopelessness, as one interviewee put it: "I became more apathetic about it. ... I stopped really caring about working to make it better. It was just kinda like well it's not gonna get better. I don't care. I'm just going to keep going the way I am. ...I didn't feel that there was anything that I was gonna [be able to do or that] it was ever going to be cured. So it was, yeah just kind of hopeless."

This is how the young man at the beginning of the chapter reached his low state: He felt like his stutter prevented him from living his life. Nothing he did seemed to make any permanent headway in achieving fluency or agency.

In a state of despair, he felt his only option was to avoid speech altogether, which destroyed his confidence and sense of self-efficacy. Plus, he knew that avoiding the problem would do nothing to solve it in the long-term; if he continued down the path he was on, he would only fall further behind his peers and his own potential.

His experience directly mirrored that of an interviewee from Corcoran and Stewart: "I was just at the end of my rope, and I just couldn't help but cry about it... I remember feeling suicidal back then and not having the courage to kill myself."

The Case for Optimism

As we plumb the depths of suffering, it's important to make clear that having a stutter does not necessarily mean that one will experience the worst of these outcomes. In contrast to the studies discussed above, research by Walter Manning and Gayle Beck found no statistically-significant differences in mental health between stutterers and fluent speakers.[16] Nor does dysfluency have to negatively affect one's life; I have met stutterers who would qualify as severely dysfluent, yet they were wonderfully content and outgoing.

I will also say, from my own anecdotal observations, that the suffering caused by stuttering seems to peak in one's early twenties. That period of life is challenging for any person; it can be overwhelming to be tossed out of the structure and social immersion of school and into the responsibility, isolation, and wide-open possibility of adult life. It seems to me that the early- and mid-twenties is a time of near-constant doubt and insecurity for many people; a speech impediment that gets worse under stress can certainly add to that.

While this darkness can seem inevitable and all-consuming, the case for hopefulness is stronger. Academic research – quantifiable, replicable research – has keyed in on treatment programs and a general "way of living" that reliably improve fluency, agency, and well-being. With these tools at hand, there is no reason for any stutterer to feel like their situation is hopeless. We cannot cure dysfluency, but everyone with a stutter should have complete confidence that they can reach their full potential and enjoy a life of thriving.

Chapter Four: Onset and Development
Why Some Children Start Stuttering and How Most Recover

While the proclivity to block is obstinately permanent in adult stutterers, the barrier between fluency and dysfluency is quite permeable in children. Of the small percentage of children who experience a period of stuttering, the vast majority make a complete recovery; their brains deviate somewhat from the normal trajectory but get back on track. That period of dysfluency may have been a stumble, but it leaves no lasting marks.

Researchers Ehud Yairi and Nicoline Ambrose estimate that about eight percent of children will experience a period of stuttering. Even though the gender ratio of adult stutterers skews heavily male, there does not appear to be a statistically-significant difference in children.[1]

Half of all cases of childhood stuttering were sudden onset: sometimes these cases were so abrupt that a child went to bed speaking fluently, but by the next morning he or she had started stuttering. The mean age of onset was thirty-three months, with sixty percent of all stutters appearing in the year between the child's second and third birthday. Eighty-five percent of all cases had manifested by the age of forty-two months, and ninety-five percent had appeared by forty-eight months. While they determined that most of the risk of stuttering has passed by the age of four, developmental stuttering can still appear through early adolescence.

It has been strongly suspected for a long time that there is a genetic component to stuttering. Children of stutterers are more likely – though not guaranteed – to have a stutter themselves. Identical twins are more likely – but not guaranteed – than fraternal twins to either both be fluent or both stutter. Research estimates that there is a 38-62% coherence between identical twins.[18]

Research in the past fifteen years has started to identify the specific genetic causes of developmental stuttering. Points of interest have been found on fourteen of the forty-six chromosomes in the human genome; six of these strongly correlated with stuttering. In addition, researchers have identified four genetic mutations (*GNPTAB*, *NAGPA*, *GNPTG*, *AP4EI*) that correlate with stuttering.[19]

It is important to point out that this research is still in its early stages. Researchers estimate that these four genetic mutations only account for 9-18% of cases of persistent adult stuttering. To date, these studies have only looked for the genetic markers that distinguish adult stutterers from adult fluent speakers; adults who recovered from stuttering in childhood were not treated as a separate cohort. Expanding the research dataset to include all people who experience at least a period of stuttering will likely increase the complexity of the findings in the future. Additionally, these results were drawn only from specific populations, like Africa and Pakistan; considering that stuttering is a global phenomenon, it's possible that its genetic sources may differ slightly depending on a person's ethnic heritage.

These findings suggest that stuttering has complex, diffuse genetic causes. Emerging research in the near future will likely uncover even more factors that contribute to stuttering. That said, there have already been some early breakthroughs in connecting the genetics of stuttering to both neurology and observable behavior.

If You Give a Mouse a Stutter...

In a 2016 study, Dennis Drayna and his team inserted a homologue of the point mutation in the *GNPTAB* gene – one of the four genetic mutations linked to stuttering – into mice. Drayna and his colleagues hypothesized that this genetic insertion could lead these mice to display vocal behaviors similar to stuttering.[20]

Why use mice in an experiment on stuttering? When separated from their mothers, mice pups will consistently and reliably call out in "bouts," crying out for a period, then going silent, then crying out again. These vocalizations have been studied and analyzed to the point that researchers can recognize the individual "syllables" in each utterance.

The mice pups who received the homologue of *GNPTAB* had noticeably different "speech" than their littermates; vocal behavior that was very similar to stuttering. They had longer gaps between bouts, suggesting they may have been experiencing hard blocks or resistance at the beginning of vocalizations. In addition, these mice had abnormal pauses during their bouts, as if they were stumbling on smaller blocks while speaking. The stuttering mice also showed less variety in their selection of syllables. Interestingly, there were no findings of repetition or prolongation blocks from the mice.

A later follow-up study, led by Tae-Un Han, examined the brains of mice who had undergone genetic manipulation in two other locations of the *Gnptab* gene.[21] These mice had developmental abnormalities in the corpus callosum like those observed in the brains of humans who stutter. Work with these mice is continuing under Shahriar SheikhBahaei, and early findings suggest that these mice have motor differences beyond vocalization.[22]

Before we go further into the neuroscience of stuttering, we need to review some basics of brain architecture.

Primer: Neuroanatomy

The brain is composed of two substances: *grey matter* and *white matter*. Grey matter composes the outer shell of the brain and, depending on its location, performs specialized, complex computations. Metaphorically speaking, grey matter operates like a computer running a particular program. Therefore, when we say that most speech processing happens in the front-left side of the brain, we are referring to the grey matter in that area of the brain.

White matter, in contrast, connects different areas of the brain; rather than performing computation itself, it passes information between regions. If grey matter is like a computer, then white matter acts as the metaphorical cables that pass data between these processing centers. These "cables," however, may sometimes be poorly connected or less capable of transmitting data than they should be.

There are two areas of the brain that are of particular importance when it comes to stuttering: the left inferior frontal gyrus and the corpus callosum. The left inferior frontal gyrus (LIFG) is situated in the left hemisphere of the brain; it's located around your temple, just behind your eye. The LIFG is home to the majority of language processing and speech production; it is also a major area of dysfunction in stutterers.

The corpus callosum is the tissue that connects the two hemispheres of the brain. While the corpus callosum's main function is to facilitate communication between the hemispheres – rather than specializing in speech – it too, has been shown to be compromised in stutterers.

Children who have begun stuttering display clear neurological differences from their fluent peers. Multiple studies have found that children who stutter have less grey matter in the LIFG, implying that they have less processing power to devote to speech. A study co-authored by Ho Ming Chow and Soo-Eun Chang found that children who stutter also had less white matter in the corpus callosum and in the left arcuate fasciculus (a white matter tract that contributes to the motor execution of speech). [23] Additionally, in two separate studies, Evan Usler, Christine Weber-Fox and Anne Smith found that stuttering children had a weaker neurological ability to perceive syntactic errors in speech, which likely cause these children to develop speech differently than their fluent peers.[24,25]

The "Cookbook" of Speech

Set aside the semantic content of speech for a moment – the thoughts, ideas, and emotions we convey with our words – and instead focus on the sound of speech itself.

Trying saying this phrase: "yee witunlob kyvustap." Even if you don't know what it means (it's pure gibberish), you can still *say* it; your brain can move your speech articulators – lips, mouth, tongue, vocal cords – in such a way that you speak each phoneme and syllable. In this context, we have removed the semantic and emotional content from speech, leaving us only with the syntactic content.

Each time you speak, your words pass through the speech sound map (SSM),† where they are translated into commands for the speech system to execute. The SSM can be thought of as a cookbook; for each phoneme in every

---

† According to the GODIVA model of speech production.[26]

language you speak, the SSM has a "recipe." This recipe – which consists of motor commands† – is passed to the speech articulators. This translation process never becomes automated; every time you speak, your speech system must look up the "recipe" for each individual phoneme. The SSM starts out blank and is gradually developed during childhood.

Children learn to speak by imitating the speech they hear from the people around them – first with incoherent screeching, then babbling, then later with sounds resembling actual language. They aim to match the speech they hear around them by using the motor commands in their underdeveloped SSM, but their imperfect productions initially miss the target. With time and practice, these "recipes" are refined until the children eventually reach the precision of adult speech.

Unfortunately, this process is hampered in children who stutter by neurological issues that are below the level of conscious attention or control. These children have an impaired ability to accurately execute speech motor commands; they are also worse at perceiving syntactic errors and errors in the audio feedback of their own speech, making it harder for them to notice and subconsciously correct imperfections in their SSM.

I will speculate that this impaired development of the SSM may be the source of the "nemesis phonemes" discussed earlier. While anxiety about a history of blocking on these phonemes may certainly contribute to increased dysfluency, there is probably a reason why these phonemes are particularly difficult in the first place. I will speculate that these phonemes do not reach full development in the SSM

_____

† The SSM also includes auditory and somatosensory expectations for each phoneme, which we will return to later.

by the end of speech development, leading the speech system to break down more frequently on these phonemes.

Recovery

Most of the 8% of children who experience a period of stuttering will make a complete recovery to perfect, effortless fluency. The figure most commonly cited for the rate of childhood recovery – 74% – comes from Yairi and Ambrose's landmark 1999 study on recovery.[27] However, that study used a relatively small number of participants and excluded the phenomenon of rapid recovery. In their 2013 study, which compiled data from multiple studies, Yairi and Ambrose updated their estimate of recovery to 91%.[1] This recovery can happen on different timelines.

A 2018 study led by Michiko Shimada observed rapid recovery in children living in Hokkaido, Japan. In Hokkaido, young children are given free-of-charge health check-ups at the ages of eighteen months and three years. Because 94.4% of the children in the city participated in these check-ups, it gave the authors incredibly reliable information.[28]

None of the children were diagnosed with stuttering at the eighteen-month check-up, primarily because their language skills were still quite rudimentary. At the three-year check-ups, however, 1.41% of the children were diagnosed with a stutter. Incredibly, when the stuttering children were brought six months later for a follow-up assessment, 82.8% of them no longer displayed stuttering.

The Shimada study had – at most – three data points when it came to the timeline of recovery. The 1999 Yairi and Ambrose study followed participants for several years, a structure that provides very specific data on the timeline of recovery. While there were participants who recovered rapidly, the more common recovery trajectory was much slower, lasting anywhere between six and thirty-five months after onset; some children even stuttered for three or four years before making a complete recovery.

Interestingly, there were clear differences between boys and girls with regards to recovery. Girls recovered at a much greater rate than boys, which explains why, despite identical rates of onset, there are three adult male stutterers for every one female. Girls also recovered earlier; peak recovery for girls was between twelve and thirty months after onset, while for boys it was between twenty-four and thirty-six months.

Regardless whether they eventually recovered or persisted, all the children showed similar levels of dysfluency at time of onset. Children whose stutter persisted showed a relatively stable level of dysfluency, though there was a slow decrease over the four years of observation.† The children who recovered, however, showed a sharp decrease in dysfluency; in fact, only one year after onset, there was already a large gap between the two groups. Similar divergence was observed in other speech metrics such as the syntactic complexity of the child's speech and the child's ability to detect syntactic errors in the speech of others. While no study suggested using these metrics as definitive indicators of future recovery or persistence, improvement at the one-year mark – or lack thereof – appeared to suggest whether or not the stutter would persist beyond childhood.[24,29]

For the most part, a stutter that persists into adolescence will likely remain permanent; however, a

---

† Yairi and Ambrose attributed some of this decrease to the fact that some children who had near-perfect fluency – who may have been considered "recovered" under less stringent criteria – were nevertheless included in the "persistent" group, bringing down the average rate of dysfluency.

study[30] published by Patrick Finn included seven stutterers who reported a complete recovery at an average age of eighteen.†

Recovery can be observed in – and likely attributed to – the resolution of the neurological anomalies that characterize stuttering. In the Chow and Chang study, all the children with a stutter lagged behind their fluent peers at time of onset in several ways: They had less grey matter in the LIFG and less-functional white matter in the LIFG and corpus callosum. However, the children who recovered caught up to their fluent peers and returned to healthy developmental trajectories; grey matter volume in the LIFG expanded to match that of fluent children, previously-impaired white matter resolved itself and passed information in a healthy manner, and their previously subpar neurological response to syntactic errors improved.

While Chow and Chang found subpar functioning of white matter across multiple areas of the brain in stuttering children, one area of particular interest was the left arcuate fasciculus; at the time of onset, all stuttering children showed decreased functionality in this white matter pathway. After recovery, the recovered children showed an increased growth rate of white matter functionality, which continued to expand at the pace recorded in fluent children. The children whose stutter persisted, in contrast, showed a *negative* growth rate in functionality. Their left arcuate

---

† While these reports are very encouraging, around that same time in my life I thought I had stopped stuttering; I've also met other stutterers who thought they recovered at that age, only to find they hadn't. Perhaps these participants made a complete recovery, or it may have been reporting error. To me, it seems likely that true recovery from stuttering – meaning the complete absence of the proclivity to block – only occurs in childhood.

fasciculus actually became less effective at transmitting signals with time, when it should have improved as they matured.

Yairi and Ambrose observed that children on the recovery trajectory never experienced a relapse; their rates of dysfluency steadily decreased over time without regression. Once the stutter had been deemed resolved, none of these children began stuttering again; they lived the rest of their lives as fluent speakers.

There is, however, at least one known way for a stutter that disappeared in childhood to re-emerge later in life. Joohi Shahed published a study on patients who had recovered from stuttering as children, only for the stutter to re-emerge, on average, six years after they were diagnosed with Parkinson's Disease. [31]

Parkinson's causes degradation of internal timing, leading to motor coordination issues – the disease's signature "tremor." Disrupted internal timing is a contributing factor in stuttering, so it follows that Parkinson's could tip a recovered brain back into stuttering.

It is important to note that this study only demonstrated that stuttering may re-emerge with Parkinson's; it did not attempt to estimate what percentage of recovered stutterers begin stuttering again when diagnosed with Parkinson's. Additionally, I have not come across any other known pathway for a recovered stutter to re-emerge, so recovered stutterers have little reason to worry.

What Separates Recovery from Persistence?

Many of these neurological insights are known thanks to a dataset collected by Soo-Eun Chang and the University of Michigan. In this research, both fluent and stuttering children had their brains scanned between two to four times over a period of several years; for the children who stuttered, scanning began as close to onset as possible.† The studies that use this data are groundbreaking for several reasons: First, they show the developmental trajectories of stuttering children as they recovered or persisted, demonstrating how the brains of these children changed as they regained fluency. Secondly, they show – reassuringly – that the brains of children who recover from stuttering differ little from those of children who never stuttered.

Furthermore, to my knowledge, the papers authored by Soo-Eun Chang, Ho Ming Chow, and Emily Garnett are the only neurological studies using data that followed participants from onset all the way to persistence or recovery. Therefore, these researchers can re-examine the children's older brain scans, knowing which of the children would eventually recover. With the power of hindsight, neurological differences from these early brain scans could help elucidate *why* some children recovered and others didn't.

Interestingly, while there were clear differences between the stuttering children and their fluent peers at the time of onset, there were hardly any observed differences between the children who would eventually recover and those whose stutter would persist. However, Chow and Chang found that while all the children who stuttered showed abnormal white matter development in the corpus callosum, the children who would recover showed less white matter connection in the front third of the corpus callosum, while the children who persisted showed

---

† The children were adequately compensated for the feat of laying still for minutes while having their brains scanned: According to the study, "All children were paid a nominal remuneration, and were given small prizes (e.g., stickers) for their participation."

abnormally high connection in the front-third, and abnormally low connection in the back two-thirds. This appears to be a very minor difference in an organ as complex as the corpus callosum, especially in a system as complex as the human brain.

Although it may seem counter-intuitive, it is very encouraging that there appears to be almost no difference between recovered and persistent children at time of onset; this implies that there may not be much separating the children who persist from those who recover. It's entirely possible that research in the near future will hone in on the key causal factors that set children on the path towards persistence or recovery; one day it may be possible to induce the recovery process in every child who begins stuttering.

But for now, what can we do for children who have started stuttering? There are speech therapy programs tailored to the needs and abilities of young children. Unfortunately, the current slate of interventions may decrease dysfluency but they do not appear to increase the odds of recovery.

Chapter Five: Childhood Treatment
Methods, Research, and Results

Children who begin stuttering are generally not distressed by it. The struggles and self-consciousness that come with stuttering generally don't arrive until adolescence. Parents, on the other hand, typically feel the stress immediately.

In a 2012 study, Laura Plexico interviewed parents of children who had started stuttering.[32] She found that parents worried that the stutter would negatively affect how other children – and the world at large – would respond to their child. Even parents who had been previously unfamiliar with stuttering could see how their child's stutter could lead to bullying, negative reactions from listeners, and a self-restricted lifestyle. Their fear was evident in the way they spoke about their children; one parent said, "I don't want him to be ostracized. That would break my heart. I don't want him to be that kid."

These parents were concerned and wanted to help, but most were uncertain how to do so. They didn't know whether simply acknowledging the stutter would be helpful or would make the stutter more intractable. They had limited knowledge about what treatment options were available and how effective they were. Most of these parents delayed treatment on advice from their pediatricians, who said that the stutter would likely pass on its own. When the stutter did not resolve after a few months, they sought help from speech therapy.

What exactly is a parent to do in this troubling situation? What treatment options are available for children who have started stuttering? And what kind of results can a parent expect from clinical speech therapy?

Treatment Options

While there are a variety of programs for childhood speech therapy, they can generally be classified into two main philosophies: "direct" and "indirect" treatment. The former directly addresses speech and the stutter, while the latter takes a more holistic approach. Both are predicated on the idea that recovery is best assisted by an increased volume of fluent speech.

The most widely-published version of the indirect approach is the "Demands and Capacities Model" (DCM).[33] The core tenant of DCM theory is that stuttering occurs when the *demands* placed on a child to speak fluently outstrip the child's *capacity* to produce fluent speech. Treatment with DCM aims to reverse that situation by decreasing the demands placed on a child by their environment and increasing the child's capacity to produce fluent speech.

For parents, time in the speech clinic is for learning to make changes to home life that are designed to increase the child's rate of fluency. A key part of this process is how the parent interacts and communicates with the child. In order to reduce demands on the child, clinicians encourage parents to speak more slowly and with more-simple language, to allow for more time between conversational turns, and to follow the child's lead during play. When clinicians work with the child, they try to reduce any stigma or emotional distress the child may be experiencing because of the stutter. While direct speech training with the child is not a required feature of DCM treatment, clinicians are instructed to use it when they feel it is appropriate.

Children are phased out of the program as their fluency improves and their speech starts to resemble that of their peers. Clinicians are encouraged to stay in touch with the family, as it is believed that major stressors in the child's life

– parental divorce, a change in school or housing, etc. – could cause the stutter to re-emerge.

In contrast, the "direct" approach focuses solely on the child's ability to produce fluent speech.

The most prominent version of the direct approach is the Lidcombe Program; this treatment program applies the Behavioral school of psychology, which became prominent in the '60s and '70s. This program's operating principle is that the stutter will be "controlled" if proper incentives and punishments are applied to the child at the correct times.[34]

At the start of Lidcombe treatment, parents are instructed in the program's signature "contingencies" – or behavioral responses – to their child's speech. Put simply, parents are told to praise their child for fluent speech, gently call attention to dysfluent speech, and intermittently remind and encourage their child to produce fluent speech. If a child stutters on a word or phrase, parents and clinicians are encouraged to ask the child to try again, under the idea that the unsatisfactory behavioral pattern – stuttering – needs to be unlearned and replaced by the satisfactory pattern of fluent speech.

As a child's fluency improves, they are moved into a maintenance phase where clinical visits and home training sessions become less frequent, eventually ceasing altogether. Should a child's fluency regress, they re-start the program.

Even when a parent is familiar with these two approaches, there are still many questions that remain. How should a parent choose between these two programs for their child? Is one program superior to the other, or do some children respond better to a particular approach?

Efficacy

While many short-term studies have been conducted on these two programs, the most complete picture comes from a study conducted by Caroline de Sonneville and Marie-Christine Franken: the Rotterdam Evaluation Study of Stuttering Therapy in preschool children – a Randomized Trial (RESTART).[35] In this study, two hundred preschool-aged children were enrolled in eighteen months of speech therapy; half were assigned to DCM and the other half were assigned to the Lidcombe Program. Results were collected after the eighteen months of treatment and again five years later. Despite the major philosophical differences between the two programs, the results were nearly identical.

In the first evaluation immediately following the end of treatment, children in both programs showed improved fluency; while the Lidcombe children showed a slightly faster decrease in dysfluency in the early months of treatment, the children's rates of fluency were roughly equal by the end of the program. Using a common metric,[†] the authors estimated that 71.4% of DCM children and 76.5% of Lidcombe children had recovered, a difference that was not statistically significant. Interestingly, the only statistically-significant difference between the two groups at this point was a slightly higher rating of quality-of-life measurement for children in the Lidcombe Program.

Five years after the end of the program, assessments of a child's recovery versus persistence could be more

---

[†] It is difficult to clearly determine whether a child has recovered from stuttering unless one is able to assess the child over several months or years. As a stand-in metric to estimate/assess a child's status, researchers record the child's speech and then count the number of dysfluencies, or "percentage of stuttered syllables" (%SS). Many studies use 2% SS as the dividing line between persistence and recovery; RESTART used 1.5% SS.

precise.[36] While parents, clinicians, and the children themselves sometimes disagreed about whether a child had recovered or not, these assessments are more reliable than those taken at the eighteen-month mark. In both programs the rate of children who were deemed recovered at the five year mark was nearly identical rate to the 1999 Yairi and Ambrose study, in which the children did not receive any speech therapy.[†]

Stuttering severity and satisfaction with speech were nearly identical between the two programs; but there were some slight differences between the two programs in the children who persisted in stuttering. The persistent children in the DCM cohort skewed more towards mild dysfluency, while there were several more "moderate" dysfluent children in the Lidcombe cohort. A greater difference was seen in quality-of-life outcomes specifically for girls; persistent girls who had gone through the Lidcombe Program had lower self-esteem and statistically significant lower self-perception of social acceptance compared to girls who persisted in the DCM cohort. This accords with anecdotes I have heard from speech therapists, that some girls will shut down emotionally or go silent when – in accordance with Lidcombe training – a speech therapist points out dysfluencies or blocks.

These quality-of-life findings make intuitive sense; should a child not recover, the holistic approach of DCM is more likely to help a child manage not only their speech but also their personal experience, whereas the sole drive of the Lidcombe Program is to remove stuttering through

---

[†] Most likely, the recovery rate in these studies was lower than Yairi and Ambrose's 2013 estimate because participants in both RESTART and Yairi & Ambrose's study had to have been stuttering for at least six months to be included. This requirement likely excluded some children who experienced rapid recovery.

conscious effort on the child's part. In addition, the parent organization of the Lidcombe Program is quite adamant that their program is effective when administered to their standards; so when a child does not recover fluency, the blame ostensibly falls on the child, their parent, or the speech therapist.

Does Speech Therapy Increase the Odds of Recovery?

Looking closely at the data, it seems that neither treatment meaningfully impacts whether a child will recover or persist in stuttering. Because the demographics of the children from the RESTART and the Yairi & Ambrose studies were very similar in terms of factors that have the greatest effect on recovery and persistence[†] we can compare across each cohort: Lidcombe versus DCM versus absence of treatment.[‡]

On average, the Lidcombe-cohort children had eighteen hours of treatment over the course of twenty-one treatment sessions, while the DCM children averaged fifteen and a half hours across seventeen sessions. Despite

---

[†] The study participants were very similar when it came to age and time since the onset of stuttering. Generally, the older a child is and the longer they have been stuttering, the lower the odds they will eventually recover. This is because children can recover anytime after onset; as time since onset increases, more children recover and leave the candidate pool, thus the ratio of children who will persist gradually increases all the way to 100%.

[‡] Lidcombe's parent organization disputed labeling the Yairi and Ambrose children as "untreated" because some of their parents were counseled one time to "reduce unnecessary pressure on the child, reduce physical and emotional excitement, and talk to the child at a slower speaking rate." What is further interesting about this counseling – and that of DCM – is that parents will often behave this way as an uncoached response to stuttering; that is, even if they never see a speech therapist.

all the effort involved in attending clinical sessions and making changes at home, these children were just as likely to recover as those who never went to a speech clinic. Based on these studies, it seems to me that the current programs likely have zero effect on recovery versus persistence.

While it's tempting to attribute a child's improved fluency to his or her time in speech therapy, research suggests that perhaps this connection is more correlation than causation. For the recovered children in the Yairi and Ambrose study, dysfluency peaked a few months after onset, then gradually decreased all the way through recovery. Several other studies found that improvement in a stuttering child's language skills over the first year of stuttering can predict recovery, even when complete cessation may not occur for another year or more.

Both DCM and the Lidcombe Program assert that relapse can occur, and if it does, treatment should resume; however, I question whether this may just be measurement error. Yairi and Ambrose observed that in their recovered cohort, there was a gradual decrease in dysfluency all the way through recovery; while fluency can vary, at no point did these children experience significant regression in dysfluency, nor did they ever relapse back into stuttering after they were deemed recovered. These sixty-two children were followed for a minimum of twelve months following recovery – some for more than four years – and *zero* of these children began stuttering again.

The neuroplastic changes accompanying recovery also dissuade me from the idea of relapse. The recovered children in these studies entered a different developmental trajectory than the persistent children; they also showed neurological development which corrected or compensated for the faults that were present at onset in all the stuttering children. While the timeline of these changes has not been teased out yet, given that eradication of dysfluency can take up to four years, I doubt that these changes occur rapidly,† or that a child may meaningfully oscillate between the persistence and recovery trajectories.

The work of Yairi and Ambrose is not the only research that raises doubts about the ability of speech therapy to induce recovery. In a state-wide survey in North Carolina, Joseph Kalinowski and Tim Saltoklarogu found very low rates of recovery for elementary school-aged children who were in speech therapy; by that age, children are unlikely to recover, so they are prime candidates for an effective intervention. The most common form of treatment for these children was two half-hourly sessions per week for several years, yet the median recovery rate reported by these speech therapists was only 13.9%, on par with what one would expect from untreated children in this age group.[37]

While speech therapy in childhood does not seem to impact recovery and persistence, it does seem that it can improve quality of life for those children whose stutter does persist. If we treat the Lidcombe cohort in RESTART as a "null treatment" in regards to mental health – it may even be a negative factor – we can see that DCM led to better fluency, self-satisfaction and perceived social acceptance for children whose stutter persisted.

If I had to suggest a course of action for a parent whose child has started stuttering, I would recommend taking the child for a speech assessment as soon as the stutter appears and then taking a follow-up assessment one year later. If a child shows meaningful improvement in fluency and the syntactic complexity of their speech over

---

† Except in rapid recovery, where stuttering lasts less than a year.

the course of that year, they are likely to recover from stuttering; as such, it seems there is not much else a parent needs to do.

If the numbers do not suggest significant improvement after a year, then the child's stutter is more likely to persist. In that case, it makes sense to enroll them in speech therapy with the aim of improving quality of life and helping them to better manage their stutter. While I see no real reason to enroll a child in a program that solely uses either "direct" or "indirect" treatment, I would strongly caution against enrolling in treatment that exclusively uses the Lidcombe Program; not only because the DCM children in RESTART had better quality-of-life metrics, but also because the studies that purport to show the infallible efficacy of the Lidcombe Program, to my mind, do not live up to the rigorous standards of peer-reviewed scientific research.[†]

I want to make it clear that my desire is not to denigrate speech therapy. I believe the primary goal of childhood speech therapy should be to increase recovery from stuttering. Improving quality of life for children whose stutter persists is absolutely a win, but if the research shows that the current speech therapy programs do not meaningfully affect recovery, we should be honest about that and adjust our expectations. Parents should not feel the need to invest so much time, effort, and hope into attaining recovery through these programs unless they are capable of delivering that effect.

[†] See Appendix: "Limitations of the Lidcombe Program and The ASRC."

Chapter Six: Neuropathology
Why The Brain Produces Stuttered Speech

I will admit this chapter is a bit bleak: Reading through a long list of cognitive deficits related to stuttering could reasonably depress someone who has a stutter. But if you have a stutter, or are sympathetic to people who do, take this as information, not a death sentence. This is the five percent of the speech system that sometimes goes wrong, not the ninety-five percent that normally goes right. And as we will see in the following chapters, researchers have found reliable paths to correcting and mitigating many of these neurological patterns. The more we know about how speech breaks down in the brain, the better equipped we are to understand and develop solutions.

The Hidden Complexity of Fluent Speech

Speech feels simple because there is little conscious attention or effort involved; you think of what you want to say, you decide to say it, and then you hear yourself say it; all of this takes place in a fraction of a second. However, the subconscious processes that produce speech are incredibly complex. Your brain performs hundreds of calculations every time you speak, drawing on multiple systems to utter the simplest phrase.

As one researcher explained, "Speech production requires the coordination of hundreds of muscles of the head, face, neck, and abdomen on a millisecond time scale, and in an overlapping manner." And that's only the physical production of speech. We also "constantly adapt to situational changes in speaking rate, articulation, and emotional load. Not only must we coordinate speech sounds like consonants and vowels, but also regulate pitch, rhythm, loudness, and prosody in order to produce natural sounding fluent speech." Humans are "nearly flawless" in our ability to handle this complex computation.[38] However, the more complex a system is, the more ways it can fail.

Plan, Execute, Monitor

Speech production is a continuous loop of three steps: *plan*, *execute*, *monitor*. In the planning phase, words are translated into motor commands for the speech articulators. Then, the articulators execute those plans in a coordinated, precise sequence. Lastly, the brain monitors feedback both to verify that speech was produced as intended and to assist in planning for the next cycle. Every sound of every syllable of every word you speak goes through this loop.[39]

Stutterers have structural and functional deficits in areas of the brain critical to this speech loop. Blocks are the tangible result of breakdowns in this invisible, subconscious process.

These deficits are spread throughout the brain and are liable to cause blocks in any phase of the speech process. Given how interdependent the phases of speech are, errors in one phase often contribute to problems in the others. Delays in the planning phase can disrupt the timing of execution. Chaotic timing during execution can prevent the feedback system from being properly cued for the monitoring phase. And weak auditory monitoring can start the next planning phase on the wrong foot.

Primer: Error-Monitoring

Before we delve into the planning and execution phases, we'll take a brief look at speech monitoring.

Whenever you speak, two separate, subconscious error-monitoring systems track your speech through feedback signals. The *auditory error map* monitors auditory feedback and the *somatosensory error map* monitors somatosensory feedback. As you speak, the error maps compare that feedback to the expectations it received from the speech sound map. When your speech feedback doesn't match expectations, the error maps fire signals to the motor cortices, which control the movement of the speech articulators. When those differences are small, the error maps will instruct the motor cortices to adjust the speech articulators in a way that will produce the desired sound. If, however, a major error is detected, the error maps will instruct the motor cortices to halt speech and start over.[26]

So, as we learn about the planning and execution phases, keep in mind that the speech system's goal is the precise and accurate execution of speech, so as not to trigger corrective error signals that can lead to dysfluency.

Phoneme Plan Selection

As discussed in Chapter Four, the *speech sound map* houses the motor commands and expectations for each phoneme in an individual's native language(s). The planning phase needs to retrieve that information, but first it must choose which phoneme to request; to do this, the speech sound map works in tandem with the basal ganglia.

The speech sound map specializes in storing and retrieving plans, not deciding which phonemes are needed. When the speech sound map processes a syllable, it sends a handful of likely matches to the basal ganglia, along with hints about which phoneme may be the best match. The basal ganglia, which is much better at selecting, chooses one, quiets the others, and sends the results back to the speech sound map. With a clear winner in hand, the speech sound map retrieves the plan and then sends commands to the motor cortices, and expectations to auditory and somatosensory cortices.

In fluent speakers' phoneme selection phase, the dopaminergic response to the winner crosses the activation threshold, while the alternatives garner little to no response. The speech sound map still has to select a match from that list, but this clear contrast in dopaminergic response makes the selection process quick and easy. Stutterers, however, have an excess of dopamine in a part of the basal ganglia called the dorsal striatum. This excessive dopamine confounds the basal ganglia's ability to select the proper speech plan for a phoneme, which was demonstrated with the GODIVA model.

The GODIVA† model is a computer program that simulates the neurological processes of speech production, from syllable selection to the movement of articulators. This program allows researchers to adjust variables to simulate how different conditions may affect the speech system. Oren Civier used the GODIVA model to simulate excessive dopamine in the basal ganglia, and found that it led to blocks.[40]

With more dopamine in play, more phonemes registered strong dopaminergic responses during phoneme selection. The best match still had the strongest response of the group, but it was no longer the clear winner; multiple phonemes crossed the "winning" threshold. This lack of a clear winner meant the speech sound map had to hold its own selection competition, an extra step that delayed the speech planning process. In the GODIVA model, this delay to the "speaker" blocking at the beginning of a phrase while it waited for the planning phase to complete.

This aberrational process could also help explain a strange phenomenon observed by Ritta Salmelin wherein a stutterer's articulators sometimes begin firing before speech

---

† Gradient Order Directions into Velocities of Articulators.

planning is even completed, something fluent speakers do not do.[41]

Incomplete Readout

In another study, Oren Civier ran the GODIVA model with parameters that mimicked the deficient white matter connection between the speech sound map and the motor cortices that has been observed in stutterers.[42] Because the simulation closely resembled the observed speech behavior of stutterers, we can use it to understand the inner mechanisms of stuttered speech.

Adults typically speak using "feedforward control," in which the speech system assumes that its motor commands have been executed properly unless the auditory feedback says otherwise. Children, however, learn to speak using "feedback control," a process in which they speak and then use auditory feedback to guide and correct their speech. Feedforward is preferred to feedback control because it is faster at responding to errors; during feedforward control, errors can be detected while the person is in the act of speaking, whereas during feedback control those errors have to be spoken and then must return back through the feedback system.

In Civier's simulations, the deficient white matter connection prevented motor commands from being transmitted as quickly and completely as they normally would be. Therefore, in order to maintain a normal speaking rate, the speech system began relying on feedback control. Because feedback control is less responsive to changes, the articulators would fall a little out of position with each transition between syllables. These minor errors accumulated over the course of an utterance, eventually reaching the point that they triggered the major errors in the error maps, causing the "speaker" to have repetition blocks.

Civier was able to observe that these repetition blocks – while disrupting fluent speech production – were actually correcting the speech errors. The "speaker" had strayed too far from the speech targets – that is, where their speech articulators should have been while they spoke the phoneme – which triggered a major error in the error maps. As the speaker repeated the syllable – "Buh-buh-buh-buh-" – Civier could see that with each repetition, the articulators were moving closer to the speech targets. Once the articulators were close enough to the target, the error maps were satisfied and speech production carried on. This repetition-until-correction mirrored behavior that has been observed in human stutterers.

In another simulation, the motor cortices were given incomplete speech plans. When this happened, the speech articulators moved into position for the first phoneme but then hung there while waiting for the rest of the motor plans to arrive. In essence, the GODIVA "speaker" was frozen with its mouth articulators in place to speak, mirroring the hard blocks seen in human stutterers.

Fundamental Motor Errors

Children speak with speech errors, but as they mature, speech production becomes more reliable and precise. Anne Smith contributed to a study which found that fluent children have greater *speech motor instability* than fluent adults.[43] The study also found that longer and more complex sentences led to more instability in fluent children, but not in fluent adults.

Anne Smith co-authored a study with Jennifer Kleinow that compared the speech motor stability of fluent adults and stuttering adults.[44] They found that the stutterers had greater instability than the fluent speakers, and that the gap was larger in sentences that were syntactically complex, but not in sentences that were simply longer. That finding suggests that the instability could be related to errors in speech planning, which is more likely to fail on syntactically-complex words. However, a group of studies conducted by Ludo Max investigated whether this motor instability came solely from errors in the planning phase.

In the first condition, fluent speakers and stutterers each read from a list of phrases while Max measured the movement of the speaker's upper lip, lower lip, and jaw.[45] There were large differences between fluent speakers and stutterers in how they performed closing movements, but interestingly, not in opening movements. Compared to fluent speakers, stutterers' movements took more time, moved more distance, and took longer to reach top speed. Max found that these differences were largest in short utterances and at the beginning of a sentence; they were smallest at the end of a sentence. Still, it was not clear whether this was the result of execution errors in the speech articulators, or if they were caused by errors during the planning phase. So, to isolate motor execution from defects in the planning phase, Max had participants make sounds completely unrelated to speech.

The participants repeated the same task, but instead of reading sentences out loud, they were given a list of non-speech facial gestures to execute, such as making a popping gesture or sticking their tongue out. Results in the non-speech task mirrored those of the speaking task: Stutterers' closing movements took longer, moved farther, and needed more time to reach top speed. These results led Max to suggest that stutterers may have a general motor deficit in the lips and jaw; even with a flawless speech plan, the motor cortices may make errors of their own.

More motor differences were found between stutterers and fluent speakers as the studies continued. Max had participants perform a task analogous to the facial movements but with their fingers. Max and his team measured the kinematics of participants while they performed varying sequences of finger movements, one of which was a finger-closing motion (picture the "come here" gesture). Even in this task, which did not involve facial movements, stutterers showed the same differences in closing movements. Max speculated that stutterers may possess a general motor deficit for closing motions, especially when initiating motor sequences.

The studies by Smith, Kleinow, and Max demonstrated motor instability in stutterers, which raises a larger question: What neurological processes are behind this behavior?

Initiating Speech

The *frontal aslant tract* in the left hemisphere of the brain is a white matter tract that connects the *left inferior frontal gyrus* to the pre-Supplementary Motor Area (pre-SMA). The left inferior frontal gyrus houses the speech sound map, and the pre-SMA's two primary roles are the initiation and coordination of sequential motor actions, such as speaking. Several studies have shown that stutterers have impaired functioning in the left frontal aslant tract.

One study in particular highlighted how impairments in the frontal aslant tract can contribute to dysfluency.[46] Dr. Rahsan Kemerdere, a neurosurgeon, wrote a retrospective of eight surgeries that removed gliomas, a type of brain tumor that lives on the outer surface of the cortex. Gliomas expand across the cortex, killing and disabling cells as they go. Since gliomas are capable of endless expansion, Dr. Kemerdere and her team aimed to excise every bit of glial tissue while leaving as much healthy tissue as possible.

All eight of her patients were confirmed to have gliomas in the frontal left hemisphere – a major speech area – but the boundaries of each glioma were unknown. In order to clearly delineate those boundaries, each patient underwent a testing phase before any brain tissue was removed.

First, the patient's cortex was exposed by removing portions of the skull while the patient was awake.† Then the patient underwent behavioral examinations while the surgical team used electrical stimulation to temporarily disable areas on the cortex. For instance, when the surgical team stimulated the primary motor area of the face, patients made involuntary facial movements. If a zap affected the patient's behavior, that part of the cortex was determined healthy and functional. If, however, the stimulation did not cause observable changes, that piece of cortex had been compromised by the glioma and would have to be removed.

Stimulation on the frontal aslant tract caused speech issues in all eight patients. None of the patients stuttered prior to surgery, but all produced stuttered speech while the frontal aslant tract was disabled. The stuttered speech resembled neurogenic stuttering rather than developmental: The proclivity to block was not affected by specific phonemes or syntactic complexity. And while speech required extra effort for the patients, none displayed secondary behaviors like eye blinking or facial grimacing.

All eight of the patients had brain matter excised during surgery, and all but one experienced issues with speech or cognition that passed with time. However, two of the patients developed a permanent neurogenic stutter as a result of the surgery. Interestingly, these were the only two patients who had their frontal aslant tracts removed.

---

† The journal article includes photos of the exposed brains, if you're curious. (And not too squeamish.)

Sequential Speech

Speech production requires two-way communication between the basal ganglia and the ventral pre-motor cortex (vPMC). At the beginning of each syllable in a word, the basal ganglia has to cue the vPMC to *start* producing the syllable. Then the vPMC has to report back that it is producing the syllable. Next, the basal ganglia has to send a cue to *stop* producing that syllable, the vPMC then reports that it has stopped producing it, and finally the basal ganglia sends a cue to start the next syllable.

This back-and-forth communication relies on the white matter fibers that connect the basal ganglia to the vPMC. Unfortunately, multiple studies have shown this connection to be relatively impaired in stutterers. When Civier ran the GODIVA model with this impaired connection, the program's basal ganglia had less context on the state of the vPMC.[40] Without timely information from the vPMC, the basal ganglia was sometimes late in cuing the vPMC to stop one syllable or start the next one. When this happened, the model would get stuck pronouncing the current syllable longer than intended. Or, in human terms, it had a prolongation block.

Timing

Speech production does not just require the coordination of hundreds of muscles; it also requires different areas of the cortex to fire at the appropriate time in order to do things like alerting the auditory cortices that speech will be coming. Getting all of these operations to fire at the appropriate time requires that they all align to a single timing mechanism. Unfortunately, that timing system can break down in stutterers, leading to blocks.[47]

The brain has two timing circuits, the *internal* and *external*. The external timing circuit aligns to external rhythms; when you nod your head to a song, that is your external timing circuit is aligning with that beat. The internal timing circuit is when the brain aligns to a signal coming from the basal ganglia.

We can see both timing circuits at work in a finger-tapping task used in research studies. The task begins with the participant listening to a rhythmic beat or a metronome. The participant taps a finger in time with the beat, aiming to exactly match the rhythm. This portion tests the external timing circuit. Then, the audio stops and the participant continues tapping, trying to maintain the same cadence as the original beat. This part of the task tests the reliability of the internal timing circuit. Stutterers perform just as well as fluent speakers when using the external timing circuit, but perform inconsistently when relying on the internal timing circuit. This discrepancy comes from a deficiency in *beta oscillations* from the basal ganglia.

Beta oscillations are brain waves seen in every part of the cortex. When these beta oscillations are in sync, separate areas of the brain can coordinate the timing of their actions. The internal timing circuit works by having the separate, disconnected areas on the cortex tune into a single set of beta oscillations coming from the basal ganglia. However, research by Andrew Etchell has found that the basal ganglia's beta oscillations are weaker in stutterers, leaving the cortex without a single, uniting signal.[48]

To understand how this would affect the ability to produce fluent speech, imagine how difficult it would be to do a jumping jack if all of your four limbs started at different times. Then think how much more complex the speech system is. Hundreds of muscles make up the speech articulators; the articulators must be in sync with each other; a breakdown in timing could lead to a logjam as breath and different muscles fire in the wrong order; or, in other words, it could cause a hard block.

Manual Connection

As Ludo Max's finger-tapping made evident, stuttering's physiological impact isn't limited to speech production. We have seen stuttering in American Sign Language, and Ludo Max showed that stutterers have a core deficiency in finger-closing movements. Now we have one more manual-language connection to explore.

Tim Saltuklaroglu conducted a circle-drawing study that showed how speech affected hand coordination in stutterers and fluent speakers.[49] Participants were asked to continuously draw a circle on a digital tablet at a steady pace under three different speaking conditions: while silent, while reading aloud, and while reading aloud in time with a partner (choral speech). Saltuklaroglu and his team then measured the "jerk" in the participants' hand movements; *jerk* was the term for deviations from the steady pace that the participants were asked to maintain.

As might be expected from the manual issues found in the Ludo Max study, stutterers had more jerk than fluent speakers in the silent condition. Additionally, speaking had no measurable effect on the fluent group, but it led to more jerk for the stutterers. During the solo speaking condition, stutterers displayed significantly more jerk than the fluent speakers.

Maybe those manual "blocks" were the result of verbal blocks; after all, they stuttered on 12% of the syllables that they spoke. However, results from the choral speaking condition shows that this is not the sole explanation. During the choral speaking exercise, the stuttering group was essentially fluent, blocking on only .3% of syllables.

However, their writing jerk was higher than in the silent condition, though not as much as during solo speaking.

This study suggests that stutterers have an impairment in fine manual control that is independent of speech, but exacerbated by speech, and especially by verbal blocks. A study by Ritta Salmelin may explain the neuroscience behind this behavioral phenomenon.

In the same study where she found that stutterers began motor activation before speech planning was completed, Salmelin also found incomplete segregation between mouth and hand motor activation.[41] Salmelin keyed in on the preparatory signals that came before motor activation. In fluent speakers, those preparatory signals were much stronger in the mouth motor cortex than in the hand areas; this makes sense, since the mouth is significantly more active during speech than the hands. Stutterers, however, displayed stronger signals in the hands than the mouth.

It is hard to know what exactly to make of that finding, but this incomplete segregation cannot help the fluent production of speech. Even prior to reading these studies, I felt like speech production was inherently more cognitively taxing for stutterers than fluent speakers. Saltuklaroglu's circle-drawing study is behavioral evidence of this, and Salmelin's finding of extraneous activation of the hands during speech may be the neurological evidence.

Motor Activation

A study led by Anna-Maria Mersov examined how motor signals may differ between fluent speakers and stutterers.[50] This study measured the *beta suppression* of participants while they read from a list of words. Beta suppression, in the simplest terms, occurs in the motor cortex during the planning and execution phases of motor movement. It can serve as an indicator for the amount of preparation and effort used in a motor movement.

Mersov found that stutterers had significantly stronger beta suppression during speech planning and motor execution than non-stutterers. This may be a result of worse speech automaticity for stutterers, which may be connected to poor speech planning. Alternatively, the stronger suppression during speech execution may be the result of weaker connections from the LIFG to the motor cortices, which has been observed in children who stutter.

Another key difference between fluent speakers and stutterers came in the silent periods between the words. After finishing one word, the *beta synchronization* in fluent speakers' mouth motor cortex returned to a resting state; it was neither preparing to speak nor resisting the urge to act. Stutterers, however showed beta synchronization between trials despite knowing they were not going to be asked to speak. Mersov theorized that stutterers' mouth motor cortices weren't fully disengaging after each trial, so extra beta suppression was required to get over that hurdle the next time they spoke. Mersov also believed this observation was connected to stutterers' deficient timing; stutterers' speech systems remained on alert because they didn't know when they would have to fire next.

The Left Auditory Cortex

Studies of the somatosensory feedback system in stutterers shows it to be functional and reliable. The auditory feedback system, however, has multiple liabilities that may contribute to dysfluency during the monitoring phase of speech.

Researcher Ritta Salmelin noted that stutterers have a "functional organization of the auditory cortex" that is "fundamentally different" than that of fluent speakers. For fluent speakers, the auditory workload is distributed between the two auditory cortices in a balanced and stable manner; however, that balance is unstable and easily disturbed in stutterers. Salmelin found that the left auditory cortex would intermittently cease processing, and the right would behave as if it was constantly loaded with feedback, even when there was little to no actual incoming sound. These issues combined to produce "transient, unpredictable abnormalities in auditory perception," undermining a key foundation in the production and monitoring of speech.[51]

In another study, Yoshikazu Kikuchi and his team found that the left auditory cortex in stutterers did not respond to repeated stimuli the same way as it did for fluent speakers. In his study, participants watched silent movies while wearing a pair of headphones. The researchers intermittently played pairs of clicks into the participants' headphones. Given that the click sounds were identical to one another and not "important," the auditory cortices of fluent speakers had a much smaller response to the second click than to the first. Stutterers, however, only showed a diminished response in the right auditory cortex; their left auditory cortex responded to the second click as if it was a novel stimulus each time. Kikuchi proposed that this inability to filter out ignorable auditory input contaminated how self-produced speech would be interpreted, leading to more errors and blocks.[52]

The Vestibular Response and Perceptual Priming

How does the brain tell the difference between the speech it hears from others, and the speech it produced itself? A key mechanism is the *vestibular response*. Vestibular mechanoreceptors, located in the ear, fire when you hear sound that is at least 70 decibels loud. They fire at a lower threshold, 35 decibels, in response to your own speech, which is detected through body vibrations. Given that speech is typically produced at 60 decibels, a vestibular response – or lack thereof – can quickly and reliably differentiate sounds as either external or self-produced.

However, research by Max Gattie has shown that stutterers had a less-sensitive vestibular response, meaning they need more audio stimulation than normal to "alert" their speech system that the voice speaking is their own. The vestibular response is a "hardware" problem that may explain a downstream "software" problem.[53]

Ludo Max and Ayoub Daliri partnered to run a series of studies about a phenomenon called *pre-speech auditory modulation* (PSAM). Like its name implies, PSAM is the phenomenon where neural activity decreases immediately preceding speech production. Max and Daliri proposed that PSAM primes the cortex to process the auditory feedback of speech in a more efficient way.

Fluent participants demonstrated PSAM both before they spoke and before they listened to a recording of themselves speaking. Stutterers, however, showed significantly less PSAM than expected in both conditions. If stutterers' auditory cortices are not sufficiently primed, they would be less capable of parsing the incoming auditory signals, which would further undermine the monitoring phase of speech.

Max and Daliri conducted this experiment again, adding a 100ms delay to the participants' auditory feedback, essentially giving them delayed auditory feedback (DAF). Interestingly, DAF had a marked effect on PSAM in both fluent speakers and stutterers. Eight of the twelve fluent speakers in that study showed *reduced* PSAM, while nine of the twelve stutterers showed *increased* PSAM that matched the levels observed in fluent speakers under normal conditions. This increased PSAM spoke well for DAF, but

Max and Daliri pointed out that the stuttering participants came to expect the delay during the course of the study, and that may have contributed to their improved fluency.[54]

Error Signals

Silvia Corbera investigated how stutterers and non-stutterers responded to auditory "errors." While participants were watching a movie, researchers would play an extra sound into the participants' headphones at regular intervals. These sounds were similar to the children's game of "duck-duck-goose" – most of the time, the researchers played the same sound (the "duck"), but at unpredictable intervals, they would play a different one (the "goose"). The unexpected "goose" sound would elicit an *auditory mismatch* signal in the participants' brains.[55]

When the researchers used basic tones – one steady sound, with deviant tones that were shorter or longer, or were a higher or lower frequency – stutterers and fluent speakers showed identical mismatch signals.

Differences emerged, however, when the tones were replaced by phonemes. In the phoneme condition, the stuttering group fired stronger mismatch signals in their left hemisphere than the fluent speakers. Interestingly, stronger mismatch signals in the stuttering group correlated with greater dysfluency.

This finding suggests that stutterers have stronger responses to auditory mismatches than fluent speakers. Even with the same level of mismatch, stutterers' error maps may fire larger error signals than those of fluent speakers, which may contribute to greater dysfluency.

This phenomenon partially explains why masking noise has been found to increase fluency; if the auditory system is liable to fire excessively-strong mismatch signals, obscuring the sound of one's own speech may make the auditory error maps less likely to fire. This could be further exacerbated by the propensity of stutterers' left auditory cortex to intermittently drop out.

Further differences emerged based on the language of the phoneme. In the second condition of the study, the participants – who were native Spanish speakers – would hear a Spanish /o/ phoneme as the "duck" sound, and either a Spanish /e/ or a Portuguese /ö/ as the "goose" sound. Corbera included the Portuguese /ö/ as a "goose" sound hypothesizing that – as a non-native phoneme that was not stored in the participants' speech sound map – the auditory cortices would process it differently than the Spanish "goose" sound.

While fluent speakers had stronger mismatch responses to the Spanish "goose" than the Portuguese "goose," the stuttering group responded identically to both of those phonemes. Corbera interpreted this outcome to mean that stutterers had difficulty discriminating native and non-native sounds, suggesting a larger issue in their ability to process all speech-like sounds.

Error Correction

The goal of the auditory error map is not to "punish" the speaker, but to correct speech execution; if an error is small enough, it can be corrected mid-speech. This functionality has been demonstrated in multiple "auditory feedback perturbation" studies.

In the first phase of a 2012 study, Shanqing Cai tested the ability of fluent speakers and stutterers to discriminate the difference in pitch between two tones. He found no significant difference between the groups in their ability to detect which of three tones were at a different frequency than the other two. This is important in light of the other half of the study, wherein both groups had to react to an unexpected change in their speech.[56]

Cai modified the way participants heard their own vowel sounds by shifting the *formant frequency* of their playback; for example, a participant may say the word "hat," but their headphones would play back "het." The participants spoke blocks of eight single-syllable words; in each block, one word would have its playback shifted down in formant frequency, and another one would be up-shifted. These unexpected shifts drew a corrective response from the participants; in response to downshifts, participants would raise the formant frequency of their speech, and they would lower it in response to upshifts.

Cai showed that stutterers were worse at correcting for these unexpected "errors." The stutterers made corrections at half the speed of fluent speakers and only corrected half as much of the error.[†] And though it did not reach statistical significance, the formant frequency of stutterers' speech was also more unstable.[57]

One particular finding from this study showed how errors in the monitoring phase can affect the subsequent planning phase: After a perturbed word, fluent speakers carried the correction into the next word; if they corrected for a down-shift on one word, they would start the next word at that adjusted formant frequency (and then correct back to baseline). This implies that the fluent speakers were able to incorporate the new auditory information into their speech plans, essentially treating it as a "new normal." Stutterers, on the other hand, did not show this effect; for better or for worse, they started each new word fresh, as if

---

[†] This was somewhat confounded by the brief nature of the stimulus. Because the stutterers corrected at a slower rate, they may have reached full correction had the target utterance been longer.

there had been no external perturbation. So, it appears the speech plans of fluent speakers were more robustly self-generated, while stutterers were "winging it" from trial to trial.[†]

Cai's study illustrates how stutterers' auditory error maps may be less able to correct errors than the maps of fluent speakers. This could be the result of any or all of the auditory issues already discussed, or it could stem from two theories suggested by Cai: First, it may be the case that the auditory error maps received incomplete or delayed expectations from the LIFG; without complete expectations in hand, it would make it harder for the auditory error map to accurately judge the audio feedback. Cai's other theory was that the auditory error maps may correctly register the errors, but their connection to the motor cortices may be flawed; a flawed connection would make it harder for the motor cortices to properly execute corrective instructions.

Because a stutterer is less able to correct errors in speech production, these errors are more likely to compound over the course of a particular utterance. If the first word is a little off-target, the next will be likely to fall even further from the goal. This theory seems to be validated by the finding that stutterers are more dysfluent on longer utterances than shorter ones.

[†] In a similar study by Cai, stutterers were also less able to correct for time-based perturbations.

A Different Cognitive Experience

Before I read these neurological studies, I thought of my stutter only in light of its most tangible aspect: dysfluent speech. Now I see stuttering as a constellation of neurological differences that change the way I perceive the world and act in it. It just so happens that some of these differences impact my ability to speak fluently. Having a stutter isn't just blocked speech; it's a completely different cognitive experience.

Reading about the effect of syntactic complexity made me re-evaluate how my stutter could affect more than just my speech. In general, I tend to communicate with syntactically-simple words. I thought I did that because simple words are more digestible. Now that I know that syntactic complexity increases dysfluency, I suspect I may have already realized this on a subconscious level and was avoiding syntactically-complex words for fear of dysfluency. Or perhaps, my aversion may come from a weakened ability to decode syntactically-complex language, even in the written word.

I was, however, quite surprised by the research on the internal timing deficit in stutterers. Music is my favorite artistic medium; I thought that if I ever played music as a hobby, I would play drums. Of the instruments that make up the prototypical rock band, I feel like my personality best matches that of drummers. Plus, I consider myself to be a pretty decent dancer, which requires rhythm.

However, since reading studies about faulty internal timing in stutterers, I've come to the conclusion that I'm not meant to be a drummer. My ability to tune into the beat of a song is rock solid, but I've since noticed that my self-generated beats quickly become inconsistent; I can be perfectly on a beat, then I'll inexplicably lose it and have to work to find it again after I've already flubbed a few beats. Still, I know of at least one stutterer who plays the drums, so it's certainly not impossible.

I'm quite surprised about Ludo Max's findings that stutterers seem to have a general motor deficit when it comes to closing motions. As an athlete, I've never felt like my hand-eye coordination was impaired in any way. However, this deficit may be contributing to my penchant to block on *cl-* and *gl-* words, and other stutterers' issues with *s-* and *p-* words, since all of those phonemes require closing motions.

I've known I had hearing issues for the past decade. Sometimes it takes an extra second after someone finishes talking for me to actually register what they said; I'll start asking a follow-up question before stopping mid-sentence and saying "...oh yeah, you literally just said that." And I'm terrible at tuning into someone's voice while in a loud environment. If I'm in a loud bar with friends, I can get by with lip reading and investing extra attention; but just as often I'll get tired, give up, and tune out while the conversation carries on without me.

Until I learned about the science behind stuttering, I thought my hearing issues came from hearing loss; after all, I've worked in loud environments, listened to loud music through headphones, and been to plenty of loud concerts. Tinnitus doesn't make everything quieter; its main effect is to reduce the clarity of your hearing – vital for listening to speech – and your ability to tune out environmental noise. It just so happens that the auditory deficits in stuttering match up perfectly with both of those symptoms. It is somewhat comforting to know that my hearing issues probably come from a genetic disorder, not poor decisions from my youth.

It also makes me think about people who have some of the developmental deficiencies of stuttering, but not all. My dad also has a hard time listening to conversations in loud environments. He also had trouble understanding me when I was a kid and spoke really fast. Now that I realize that stuttering does not have any one single cause, and in light of my genetic connection with my father, I wonder if some people have *some*, but not *all* of the pathologies that cause stuttering. They may have poor diction, or issues processing rapid speech, but not the "critical mass" that creates the propensity to block.

Similarly, I wonder if all of the neurological differences above contribute to stuttering. Perhaps each of these deficits contributes to the network effect that leads to stuttering. Or it may be the case that developmental stuttering only requires a few key causal differences. After all, it seems that the patients in the Kemerdere study developed a neurogenic stutter solely because their left frontal aslant tracts were removed. Therefore, it may be the case that some of these differences are "silent failures" that don't actually contribute to stuttered speech. That would be great news, because it would reduce the neurological distance between stutterers and fluent speakers, requiring fewer neurological changes to cure a stutter that persisted to adulthood.

Neuroplasticity: The Saving Grace

It can be difficult to digest the deep-seated nature of stuttering's neurological roots, but there is also good news.

Everything covered in this chapter is a neurological deficit that has been demonstrated in rigorous scientific studies, but that doesn't mean they are life sentences. The brain can compensate for deficits in one function by recruiting other areas of the brain or by strengthening supporting areas in a process called *neuroplasticity*.

The core pathologies of stuttering can lead the brain to produce neuroplastic adaptations in a haphazard way, a response which correlates with the most severe dysfluency. However, multiple studies have shown that speech therapy produces guided adaptations that reliably normalize maladaptive patterns and increase fluency.

Chapter Seven: Speech Therapy and Neuroplasticity
Changing Fluency by Changing the Brain

Every stutterer knows that fluency can change over the course of one's lifetime, but not everyone understands why. For stutterers and non-stutterers alike, the brain changes in a process called *neuroplasticity*. When we consider that blocks are the end result of breakdowns in the speech system, it begs the question: Are neuroplastic changes connected to these changes in fluency? And if that's the case, could we harness neuroplasticity in a way that reliably improves fluency?

Unguided Adaptation

Children who persist in stuttering travel down a different developmental trajectory than their fluent or recovered peers, leading to a host of neurological differences between themselves and fluent speakers in adulthood.

However, these neurological differences can further diverge as the brain responds to the etiological origins of the disorder, almost as if the brain is consciously seeking ways to counteract dysfluency. When the brain does this of its own accord, it is called *unguided adaptation*.

There are unguided adaptations that increase fluency, but there are also those that actually exacerbate the core etiology of stuttering. Like an athlete compensating for weak legs by lifting with their back, sometimes these "fixes" further destabilize the system.

One example of this phenomenon is the balance between auditory and somatosensory feedback. From late childhood onwards, the speech system prioritizes auditory feedback, while somatosensory feedback is secondary. However, stutterers have errors in processing auditory information, resulting in inconsistent auditory feedback and delayed auditory processing. In response to this aberration, some stutterers' brains compensate by placing more emphasis on somatosensory feedback, to the point that it takes precedence over auditory feedback. This is less than desirable because auditory feedback is processed faster and helps with the timing of speech production.[26,40,42,58]

I will speculate that unguided maladaptations like these are the primary cause of severe dysfluency, not because an individual has a more severe etiology, or a "worse" stutter. I say this because there are interventions that simultaneously normalize unguided adaptations and improve fluency. In other words, when a stutterer's brain is returned to its "default state," dysfluency becomes mild.

Normalization Through Speech Therapy

Speech therapy yields different results for different people: Some swear that it was a turning point in their life while others saw no real or lasting improvement.

Many stutterers who go to speech therapy do so on a weekly basis; during these sessions, they learn and practice a set of fluency-inducing techniques. These techniques are often taught as mitigation techniques, meant to be used to work through blocks in the real world. While these techniques may help stutterers prevent or work through blocks, they also sound unnatural and require deliberate effort, so it is difficult for stutterers to consistently use them. These techniques also require conscious attention, so they cannot become a default way of speaking. Performing these exercises for several hours at a time, however, drives neuroplastic change that correlates with higher rates of fluency.

Intensive speech therapy – that is, several hours of speech therapy a day for one-to-three weeks – has been found to be quite effective in improving fluency in a very short period of time. In the dozens of studies that I have read on speech therapy, most participants began their program with a percentage of stuttered syllables (%SS) in the middle single-digits – which would be considered moderate dysfluency. However, nearly every participant – even those who started at 23% SS – finished at 2% SS, which would be considered mild dysfluency, by the end of the program.† Additionally, in a study by Katrin Neumann, participants also finished speech therapy with better control of their vocal cords and more dynamism in their speech.[59,60]

Researchers have found that intensive speech therapy results in more than just improvements in fluency: It produces neuroplastic changes as well. Christian Kell observed "profound changes" in the way his participants activated their speech networks as a result of speech therapy. Before the therapeutic program, connectivity within the left hemisphere of his participants' speech networks was "remarkably different" than that of fluent speakers, but these differences were "largely attenuated" after therapy.[61]

At a detailed level, Kell observed that the connection between the auditory and motor cortices had been improved, leading to better processing of auditory input. With auditory information re-incorporated into the speech system, the over-reliance on somatosensory feedback was normalized, and the auditory-somatosensory balance was

---

† To put that figure into perspective, the speech of fluent speakers tends to be scored around .6% SS.

once again tipped in favor of auditory feedback, as it is in fluent speakers.

Anne Giraud authored a study that highlights speech therapy's ability to undo maladaptations and reduce neurological differences between fluent speakers and stutterers. She found that, prior to speech therapy, some of her participants had excessive activation in the *caudate* – a section of the basal ganglia – but other participants had unusually low activation in the same area. Interestingly, after speech therapy the over-activators showed less caudal activation than they had before, while the under-activators had greater activation; although speech therapy affected each group differently, it brought both groups back to the levels seen in fluent speakers.[62]

Speech therapy can change the brains of stutterers for the better, but how does it do that? After all, the therapeutic programs used in these studies were not developed in response to the findings of modern neuroscience. The treatment guide for Fluency-Shaping Therapy, the core philosophy of modern speech therapy, was first published in 1975, but nearly every neurological study mentioned in this book was published after the year 2000.[63]

One clue to this puzzle comes from the GODIVA computer model, which allowed Oren Civier to peek inside the speech system while it performed speech therapy techniques.

Why It Works

As discussed in the previous chapter, Civier induced the GODIVA model to "stutter" when – in imitation of stutterers' speech systems – he weakened the program's speech motor control and delayed its processing of auditory feedback. Impaired speech control caused the model to miss its speech targets, and the delayed processing of auditory feedback prevented the auditory error maps from recognizing and correcting for those errors. Therefore, as the model moved from phoneme to phoneme and syllable to syllable, its pronunciation errors compounded until the model was so far off its speech targets that it triggered repetition blocks.[42]

Civier ran the model again with the same neural parameters, but this time he had it mimic a speech therapy technique called "elongated syllables," which has been known since the 1950s to induce near-perfect fluency. To practice this technique, the speaker slows their rate of speech by holding each syllable for twice as long as normal.

When the GODIVA model spoke with elongated syllables, the slower rate of speech created more time for auditory processing to occur, which then enabled the incorporation of auditory feedback into speech production. With auditory feedback re-incorporated into the speech system, the model could recognize and correct for minor errors in motor execution. Additionally, with more time for the articulators to produce each syllable, the model was significantly more capable of reaching the full and accurate expression of each phoneme. This in turn led to more accurate transitions between syllables, which resulted in increased fluency.

Elongated syllables increased the neurological connection to auditory feedback while it's being used, but it may also drive the long-term re-incorporation of auditory feedback into speech. Kell noted that while his participants were deficient at detecting rapid changes in speech sounds, they had a healthy ability to detect slow changes. Perhaps elongated syllables helped the brain pick up auditory feedback again, and intensive practice may have trained the speech system to re-incorporate auditory feedback into speech production.[61]

Kell also postulated that slowing down speech to produce elongated syllables requires the speaker to be more conscious of speech timing, which may counter potential negative effects of the internal timing deficit.[58]

Why It Matters

Taken together, these studies paint a clear picture: Dysfluency can be exacerbated if the brain adapts to stuttering in an unhelpful way. Fortunately, intensive speech therapy can improve fluency by removing these maladaptations and bringing stutterers' speech systems closer to those of fluent speakers. This treatment effect is true for any stutterer, regardless of their initial level of dysfluency. This offers a tremendous window of hope for all stutterers.

We've reached a turning point. Now we will shift from what a stutter *is*, to *what we can be do about it*: the specific programs you can use to increase fluency, live with greater agency, and reach your full potential. The research has provided us with the path; all that's left is to put in the work.

Chapter Eight: The Gameplan
How to Improve Fluency and Quality of Life

Earlier chapters established how stuttered speech is the result of pathology in the brain's speech system. We also saw that the brain can respond to this neuropathology with patchwork adaptations that actually destabilize the speech system and exacerbate dysfluency. However, intensive speech therapy can increase fluency by removing those maladaptations and routing speech through default pathways.

Now it's time to turn the scientific research into a real-life, actionable plan: to either make the most of a speech therapy experience or use an equally-effective self-directed program. This chapter also addresses mental health since anxiety disorders and avoidant behavior patterns can prevent stutterers from utilizing newfound fluency.

This information can guide us on a journey out of suffering and into liberation.

Speech Therapy

To best replicate the neuroplastic improvements observed in studies led by Gordon Blood, Luc De Nil, Christian Kell, and Katrin Neumann, we should aim to replicate their interventions.[58,59,60,64]

It's important to note that these studies used intensive programs – multiple hours per day for two-to-three weeks – yet many stutterers seeking treatment attend only one speech therapy session per week.

While I did not find any studies on the neuroplastic effects of weekly sessions, research on other disorders has shown that weekly programs produce less neuroplastic change than intensive ones; in other words, fifty hours of therapy over three weeks will be more effective than fifty hours spread over five months. These findings suggest that stutterers who are not satisfied with their progress in weekly sessions should consider switching to an intensive program.[65]

Most intensive speech programs largely follow the same patterns and use the same tried-and-true exercises as one another. The program used in Gordon Blood's study does not represent the totality of treatment, but it serves as a good example.

Participants in Blood's study progressed through the treatment program depending on their ability to successfully complete the curriculum of speech exercises. It took participants about fifty hours to complete the program, split into three or four sessions a week for three weeks. These exercises rebuilt speech motor execution from the ground up by removing bad habits and then exaggerating fluency-inducing aspects of speech.

After secondary behaviors – like eye blinks, fist clenching, and facial grimacing – were unlearned, participants learned new breathing patterns. They trained producing a steady stream of air – first in isolation, then while speaking. They also practiced gentler transitions between syllables through easy onsets to speech and worked on maintaining phonation through the entirety of an utterance. Participants mastered these components in isolation before learning to apply them all simultaneously. This manner of speech, while more fluent, also sounds unnatural; so, the final stage was to sound more natural while applying these techniques.

After completing this intensive program, participants enrolled in a maintenance program.

Interestingly, speech therapy can be delivered in a variety of ways. Traditionally, a speech therapist would teach a client these techniques, practice them with the client, and then deliver feedback and coaching on the client's execution. This was the method used in De Nil's study. However, speech therapy can also be delivered through computer programs, as was the case in the studies of Blood, Kell, and Neumann.

Computerized programs typically rely on a microphone (and in some cases a respiratory sensor) to gauge whether the client performed a technique correctly. After the participant successfully hits the specified targets for the technique a predetermined number of times, the program advances to the next task.

It's incredible to me that computer programs can effectively deliver speech therapy with little to no personal coaching. Blood's 1995 study produced incredible results even though the technology of that era was quite rudimentary compared to modern computing. If a computer running on the MS-DOS operating system was able to deliver a complete speech therapy program, it's reasonable to believe that a smartphone app could do the same. Therapy-seekers would still need the self-discipline to commit up to fifty hours over three weeks, but this easy and cost-effective access to treatment is incredibly exciting.

These studies also show the importance of enrolling in a maintenance program after completing the intensive portion of therapy. Maintenance programs protect against the potential for fluency gained in the clinic to not translate to the real world. Furthermore, Neumann showed that neuroplastic improvements continued to mature over the course of the one-year maintenance program. While we do not yet know whether it's necessary to be in a maintenance program to realize those maturations, it almost certainly doesn't hurt.

In Blood's study, maintenance sessions began with a fifteen-minute refresher on the computer program, followed by thirty-five minutes of cognitive-behavioral counseling. Counseling focused on the personal side of stuttering management; topics such as attitude change, relapse management, self-esteem, self-responsibility and coping skills.

Blood's participants completed three maintenance sessions a week for six-to-eight months. De Nil's maintenance program required fewer hours than Blood's but was equally effective. His participants had one session every week for the first month, then one every other week during the second month, and then one session per month for the final ten months.

It's important to acknowledge that not everyone with a stutter will have both the resources and the desire to enroll in an intensive clinical program. For that reason, it's worth examining some alternatives to clinical speech therapy. These self-directed programs increase fluency and drive many of the same neuroplastic changes as traditional interventions, but they can be done independently and at little-to-no cost.

Self-Directed Speech Therapy

If practicing speech therapy's tried-and-true fluency-inducing techniques for dozens of hours stimulates neuroplastic change, could stutterers achieve similar results using other fluency-inducing techniques?

Earlier, we showed that faulty internal timing is one of the neuropathologies that contributes to stuttering. The brain needs steady timing to coordinate the actions of individual components in complex processes like speech production; this timing can come from the external timing circuit or the brain's internal timing circuit.

However, the internal timing circuit of stutterers is compromised by too-weak beta oscillations in the basal ganglia. These intermittent failures in the timing circuit are liable to disrupt the smooth production of speech, resulting in blocks and dysfluency.

Stutterers have a healthy external timing circuit, though, which explains why stutterers are significantly more fluent when timing their speech to external cues like music or a metronome.[47]

If metronomic speech is a fluency-inducing technique, could consistent training with it increase fluency and drive neuroplastic change? This was directly investigated by Jean Paul Brady in 1971 and Akira Toyomura in 2015.[66,67]

The structure of the training programs used by the two researchers were slightly different, but participants in both studies improved their fluency. All of Toyomura's participants – regardless of their initial levels of dysfluency – qualified as mild stutterers by the end of the metronome regimen. Some of Brady's participants still had moderate dysfluency, but those were the same participants with the most severe dysfluency at the start of the program. Brady suggested that the most severely dysfluent stutterers might consider wearing a metronomic device in their ear, similar to a hearing aid. These participants reported that the minor inconvenience of wearing such a device was worth the drastic improvement in their fluency.

In an earlier study, Toyomura had shown that the basal ganglia activation of stutterers lagged behind fluent speaker during self-paced speech, but metronomic speech brought those levels up to parity.[68] Toyomura's 2015 study showed that consistent metronome training made the temporary benefits of metronomic speech more permanent; activation in the participants' basal gangliae increased to match that of fluent speakers even during self-paced speech. Toyomura also found decreased activation in the cerebellum, implying less of a need to correct motor execution and timing. While beta oscillations were not measured, we can reasonably infer that their volume increased as well.†

Though both studies centered on metronomic speech practice, this was achieved in slightly different ways. Toyomura's participants were instructed to read aloud to a metronome for at least fifteen minutes a day, at least five days a week, for eight weeks. Participants who did longer or more frequent sessions saw greater gains. Brady's program was structured more like traditional speech therapy; once Brady trained participants on how to use the metronome, they were expected to practice metronomic speech for forty-five minutes a day for the first two-to-four weeks. As this intensity tapered off, Brady then asked his participants to incorporate metronomic speech into their daily lives, whether through conversation with family members and friends or by reading aloud with those people as an audience. Once his subjects saw improved fluency and comfort with using metronomic speech in training sessions, they began using it in the real world.

Interestingly, the two studies also put forth different philosophies for progression as participants became more competent with metronomic speech. Toyomura instructed his participants to always speak one syllable per beat but to increase the speed of the metronome as they improved. Participants typically started with the metronome at around

---

† According to Andrew Etchell.

90 beats per minute but progressed to around 120 beats per minute by the end of the program. It's interesting that the participants' speech naturalness improved, despite this somewhat-rigid speaking pattern. This is also exciting, considering that clinical speech therapy usually leads to a temporary drop in speech naturalness.

Brady took a different approach to progression; instead of speeding up the beat, his participants spoke more syllables per beat. Brady encouraged them to speak two syllables per beat, then to fit entire phrases and even sentences into a single beat. He also taught participants to better mimic the flow of natural speech by occasionally skipping a beat. Unfortunately, Brady did not measure speech naturalness in his study; however, since naturalness improved in Toyomura's study – where speech patterns were more rigid – I believe we can expect that Brady's participants also made gains in speech naturalness.

Toyomura's program ended after eight weeks of at-home training, but Brady's program had real-world application built into it. Participants made a ranked list of challenging speaking situations and then practiced taking them on. To ease them into each situation, participants first practiced these real-life scenarios with the metronomic device playing in their ear, as a sort of lifeline. As they became more comfortable and fluent, they gradually decreased their use of the device, eventually speaking exclusively without it. Brady advised his participants to return to metronome training when they experienced drops in fluency; he reported that these recovery sessions usually corrected potential relapses after only a few days.

Brady's study included follow-up measurements for each participant. While the timing of follow-up differed between participants – fourteen months on average, but ranging from six months to four years – almost every participant not only retained their therapeutic gains, but continued to improve even after the program ended. Toyomura's study concluded at the end of the training program, so unfortunately we don't know if these neuroplastic changes endured, or for how long. However, in light of how well fluency was retained by Brady's participants, I believe we can reasonably expect the neuroplastic changes to have also lasted for a long time.

These programs are an incredible boon to stutterers given how simple and accessible they are. Metronomes are relatively cheap, and many websites offer metronomic functions for free. That means there are almost no barriers to stutterers implementing these programs in their own life.

Another self-directed program can be developed from research conducted by Chunming Lu. His intervention was somewhat particular to languages like Mandarin Chinese, which are written in pictographic characters. That said, I believe the principles are broad enough that we can adapt aspects of his program to benefit anyone with a stutter. One can suppose that, even for native speakers, translating pictographs into syllables and phonemes adds an extra cognitive step to speech production. Therefore, Lu investigated whether fluency could be improved by making the phonetic content of words more obvious.[69]

Lu's participants completed an intensive seven-day program that focused on the recitation of syntactically-simple words; each word was composed of only two syllables, and each syllable followed a consonant-vowel pattern (such as *baby*, *busy*, *dizzy*). In the first of three daily training sessions, the participant worked through a list of these words with a diction expert; the diction expert recited each word twice, and then the participant recited it back twice. In the following two sessions, the participant read aloud from the wordlist by themselves. In the read-aloud sessions, the words were printed in Pinyin Chinese, since this spelling is more phonologically transparent. In Pinyin, words are written in Roman characters instead of pictographs; for example, the word for "building," 建築, would be written as "jiàn zhú."

There was always a speech therapist present during training sessions, but the therapist did not provide feedback until the end of each day, at which point the speech therapist and participant would discuss the speaker's performance. As in Brady and Toyomura's programs, participants were encouraged to apply strategies from the study when they encountered dysfluency in real life.

At the end of the program, participants had fluency gains matching those of traditional clinical programs. Additionally, brain scans of the participants showed increased activation of the LIFG and decreased cerebellar activation, similar to the effects of traditional speech therapy. Lu conducted this intervention twice, using different scanning technologies, and found similar neuroplastic improvement both times.[70]

How can we adapt this program to languages that do not use pictographic characters while still retaining its effectiveness? We don't have enough information to pinpoint the exact causal mechanism(s) of Lu's program, but the two most salient factors appear to be the conversion to Pinyin spelling and the intensive recitation of syntactically-simple words. In the absence of studies that separate the two components, we can't confidently determine how much each one contributed to the program's success. However, I believe that one could gain most of the neuroplastic changes and improved fluency of Lu's program by reciting syntactically-simple words for several hours a day.

It seems to me that syntactically-simple words are a great training tool for independent speech practice. Stutterers are more fluent than normal when reciting syntactically-simple words. Many repetitions of highly-fluent speech – proper executions of the speech system – could drive corrective neuroplastic change in adult stutterers; this practice would function like intensive speech therapy, but without traditional fluency-inducing techniques.

However, reciting simple words for several hours a day would likely be painfully monotonous and thus difficult to sustain on one's own. So I propose a practice that may be more amenable: reading aloud.

All you have to do is take out a book you enjoy, go someplace where you have a reasonable amount of privacy, and read aloud for twenty minutes.

Reading aloud gives you limitless material with which to practice your speech. It also removes all effort and attention from *what* to say and allows you to focus solely on *how* you say it. By doing this in the privacy of your own home, you can mindfully notice what strategies allow you to work through blocks when you encounter them. (And enjoy some good books in the process!)

From my own experience, after ten minutes of reading aloud, I've lost whatever self-consciousness or anxiety I started with. I usually stop after twenty minutes due to mental fatigue; at that point, my brain feels spent, but it also seems like it's operating more effectively. Subjectively, my baseline fluency also feels improved afterwards.

This reading doesn't need to be dry or monotonous; in fact, more emotive reading will likely be more effective. In her work on stuttering and prosody, Neumann noted that emotional and linguistic prosody activate the LIFG more than flat, affectless speech. She posited that speaking with prosody could further stimulate the neuroplastic healing of white matter connections in the LIFG. Therefore, if you practice reading aloud, it would be most beneficial to speak with emotional affect and flow with the rhythm of the writing.[60]

I often practice reading aloud when I have an important or stressful speaking situation on the horizon. Even though my fluency is usually pretty good and I'm relatively comfortable in those situations, I still get jitters. I think of it like an athlete warming up before a game: Reading aloud doesn't guarantee fluency in the live scenario, but it does better prepare me for success. I also use this practice if I've gone a few days without much social interaction and my speech system feels rusty. Reading aloud is an easy and accessible way to loosen the gears and get over the mental hurdle of returning to speech. Alternatively, I'll use reading aloud to counter a relapse in fluency, similar to the way Brady's participants used metronome refreshers.

Be deliberate with the reading material you select; choose something that you enjoy and expect to make you feel better. Personally, I like reading essays by Ralph Waldo Emerson, because I find his work enlightening and inspiring. After twenty minutes of reading Emerson, not only have I exercised my speech system and improved my fluency, I'm also in an elevated state of mind.

Avoiding speech for fear of stuttering undercuts a person's self-confidence and sense of agency. If we are to mitigate the totality of a stutter, we should not leave this unresolved.

The Personal Side of Recovery

Speech therapy can greatly improve fluency, but subjective well-being for stutterers is not strictly tied to dysfluency. Therapeutic goals can be just as much about taking back control of one's life as it is about stuttering less. Similarly, does better fluency necessarily lead to greater agency and well-being?

A 2008 study led by Ross Menzies investigated the connection between improved fluency and overall quality of life. In this study, all elements of real-world application and cognitive-behavioral change – which are typically part of speech therapy – were removed. This boiled down the therapeutic program solely to training and practicing speech motor correction.[71]

Participants were given a battery of assessments at different stages of the study. In addition to measuring fluency, participants were assessed on mental health, well-being, and agency. One assessment was specifically designed to measure the participants' ability to take on difficult speaking situations. Before therapy began, participants made a list of ten challenging speaking situations, ranked them from easiest to most difficult, then indicated the most difficult task they would be willing to do.

This stripped-down therapeutic program produced fluency gains commensurate with full clinical programs of the same duration, and a one-year follow-up found that participants maintained their improved fluency.[†] In general, assessments suggested that the participants' mental health was slightly better immediately following the end of the program, and it had improved further by the one-year follow-up. With each successive measurement, participants

---

[†] Participants were offered maintenance sessions, but it was not indicated how many took advantage of that opportunity.

increased the number of tasks they were willing to perform. However, their rates of social anxiety did not change, even after living with improved fluency for an entire year.

These results show that improved fluency by itself will not resolve the suffering and limitation caused by stuttering. Participants were significantly more fluent after this clinical program, yet stuttering was still a major mental obstacle and source of distress.

Fortunately, these participants were only one half of a split-cohort study. The real intention of the study was to isolate the effects of cognitive-behavioral therapy (CBT) on clinical speech therapy. This first group was the "control" group; they showed the efficacy of speech therapy when all cognitive-behavioral elements were removed. The other half of participants, the CBT cohort, provided insight into how CBT can affect agency, well-being, and fluency.

The CBT cohort completed ten weekly sessions of CBT before speech therapy began. This by itself produced immediate benefits for the participants' mental health; gains that were roughly equal to the control group's cumulative improvement at the one-year follow-up! With no changes to their fluency, the CBT cohort was willing to take on 90% of challenges from their task list, up from 30% at first measurement. For comparison, at their best, the control group participants were willing to do 65% of the items on their task lists.

From this data, it is clear that the CBT group began speech therapy in a much better state of mind. Interestingly, the two cohorts showed only minor differences in fluency throughout the course of the program. The CBT cohort's well-being and agency, however, was improved at the end of speech therapy and had improved even further by the follow-up measurement. Immediately after therapy and at the one-year follow-up, most of the CBT group members were willing to complete every item on their challenge list.

The clearest difference between the groups, however, was in their rates of social anxiety. Throughout the entire course of the study, the control group remained at a 50% diagnosis rate. Half of the fourteen CBT participants were diagnosed with social anxiety at intake, too, but at follow-up that number was *zero.*

Menzies' study suggests that CBT (and similar mental health interventions) could directly address the high prevalence of distress and mental health disorders in stutterers. That the CBT cohort saw major gains in agency even before starting speech therapy shows that, no matter how dysfluent someone may be, they don't need to be limited by distress and anxiety.

Cognitive-behavioral therapy pairs so well with speech therapy because it helps participants put their newfound fluency into action. In fact, it's critical to change attitudes and habits – and not just speech patterns – in order for improved fluency to have a meaningful impact on your life.

For contrast, a study led by Lisa Iverach shows what can happen to fluency if behavior patterns and mental health diagnoses are left unresolved. Iverach's participants completed a week-long intensive clinical program followed by seven weekly maintenance sessions. All participants had improved fluency at the end of the intensive program, but at six-month follow-up, only one-third had retained their gains; the rest regressed about halfway back to their original levels of fluency. To be fair, the therapeutic program was relatively short, and the maintenance program did not seem to be as rigorous as the others we've seen. This shorter program could be a contributing factor to the relapse, but when we look at the participants' mental health, the picture becomes clearer.[72]

The participants completed a mental health questionnaire before the start of the therapeutic program. This questionnaire placed emphasis on anxiety disorders and how often participants avoided or withdrew from stressful situations. The two-thirds of the cohort that relapsed all qualified for at least one mental health diagnosis, while the one-third without any diagnoses retained their fluency. To further demonstrate the effect of mental health, those with two or three diagnoses lost more fluency than those with only one.

It can be inferred from this data that the two-thirds who relapsed had difficulty utilizing their new fluency in the real world. Even though speech therapy made them more likely to be fluent, they continued to avoid stressful speaking situations. This study hammers home an important point: If you do not use your new fluency, you lose it.

Successful speech therapy therefore demands cognitive-behavioral change and real-world application. Menzies' study in particular highlights why these elements are typically included in speech therapy and why they are so important. For these reasons, it would be wise to ensure that your speech therapy program incorporates elements of cognitive-behavioral therapy.

These studies also show that relatively-good fluency does not necessarily protect from the distress and limitations of stuttering. If your dysfluency is mild but you are still suffering, you may want to consider enrolling in a cognitive-behavioral therapy program.

If you are going the way of self-directed speech therapy, consider working with a CBT professional to assist you in maintenance and real-world application. However, not everyone has the time, resources, or interest in this professional support; therefore we'll take a look at what a self-directed application and maintenance program may look like.

Self-Directed Application and Maintenance

Cognitive-behavioral therapy works by helping clients modify behavioral patterns and correct cognitive distortions. It's a broad philosophy with many useful strategies and techniques, but we'll focus on two tools that are particularly applicable to stuttering.

The first is *systematic desensitization*, a process in which the participant deliberately exposes themselves to scary situations in order to expand competence. When systematic desensitization is used properly, participants can gradually develop the attitude, fortitude, and competence to regularly do things that used to scare them.

You can guide yourself through systematic desensitization by adapting a procedure used in the work of Brady and Menzies. Write down between ten to twenty difficult speaking situations, and then rank them from easiest to hardest. Figure out which ones you are reasonably comfortable doing, and then push yourself into a situation that is just one ranking more difficult. Take the challenge on, even though it's uncomfortable, or a bit scary. Each time you do that task, it will become less stressful, less fear-inducing. Eventually, that task will not be particularly challenging; you'll become confident and competent when doing it. Once you reach that point, take on the next item from your list.

This is all the strategy and technique you need; achieving progress only requires you to supply the discipline and commitment to sustain this practice.

Doing something outside your comfort zone is – by definition – uncomfortable, and you will likely be dealing with stress when it comes time to act. This can lead to anxiety, and your mind conjuring vivid worst-case scenarios. If you have a stutter, you may worry that you will block, that you will embarrass yourself, that people will laugh at you. To be fair, those are all valid possibilities. They could realistically happen.

Your anxious brain may try to convince you that these worst-case scenarios *will* happen, but the truth is that you really can't know until you try. If reality turns out any better than your worst fears, your anxiety will have done you a disservice. If that is the case, you would benefit from training yourself to set better expectations. To help manage the stress and anxiety that comes from pushing boundaries, we turn to our next CBT tool: *behavioral experiments.*

If you record your expectations before entering a situation, you can compare them to the actual outcome after the fact. The attempt may turn out really well. It might end up quietly neutral. Or perhaps it does go poorly, but not nearly as painful as you feared. If you record and compare your expectations often enough, it becomes easier to put anxiety into perspective and to recognize exaggerated worries for what they are. With that information, you can set more reasonable expectations in the future.

In those moments when your brain is conjuring up all kinds of terrible outcomes – when you can see yourself blocking and getting laughed at – mentally take a step back and remind yourself "I've felt this way before. And nearly every time, it didn't go as poorly as I feared. Even when it did, the reality of the outcome was often not as bad as I had feared." With time and practice, you will learn to calm down, contain the anxiety, and detach from the stress of the situation.

Another strategy for detaching from a chaotic internal experience is *mindfulness*; which is, in my opinion, one of the best tools for the lifelong management of a stutter. We know that fluency varies with your internal state; good internal states typically lead to better fluency, and bad ones lead to worse dysfluency. Combining my personal experience with the neuroscientific literature, I will posit that once the neurological maladaptations of severe dysfluency have been normalized, the greatest potential gains lie in managing one's internal state. And while it is impossible to always be in good states and to never be in bad ones, mindfulness can help you encourage the former and let go of the latter. The detachment from internal experience that comes with mindfulness practice can function in much the same way as behavioral experiments.

Mindfulness gives an increased awareness of your own internal state and the ability to strategically detach from intense emotions. With practice, you can take a mental step back from stress and instead think "Ah, I am feeling anxious about this situation. Because I am anxious, my expectations are likely to be unrealistically negative. Therefore, I should not place too much stock in these predictions." As your practice develops, you learn to not only notice your internal state, but also to gently guide it; therefore, you could learn to let go of the nervousness you were feeling and instead stay calm and centered on the task at hand.

Meditation may also help mitigate some of the neuropathology of stuttering, as was shown in a 2019 study by Daiki Miyashiro. Recall that delayed audio feedback (DAF) paradoxically makes stutterers almost perfectly fluent but causes fluent speakers to stutter. In Miyashiro's study, a cohort of fluent speakers spoke under DAF while researchers recorded the fluency of their speech and their neurological responses to audio. For the next eight weeks, half of the participants meditated everyday for ten minutes, and then the entire group was scanned again while they had DAF playback in their ears. The control group showed the same dysfluency as in the first trials, but the meditation group showed greater fluency and better neurological responses.[73]

Miyashiro posited that the meditation group was better able to allocate their attention, and thus could ignore audio feedback that would normally make them stutter. This effect would be helpful for stutterers because blocks can be caused by problems with parsing audio feedback and incorporating it into speech production. Additionally, one can optimistically suppose that – whatever the causal mechanism may be – if mindfulness enabled fluent speakers to be more fluent under DAF, it may help stutterers be more fluent in our "normal" circumstances.

Lastly, I believe that stutterers would benefit from processing their own feelings about stuttering. Let's be honest: having a stutter sucks. The reality is that having a stutter – even one that is well-managed – is objectively worse than not having a stutter. We may tell ourselves that the stutter isn't that big of a problem, but it's still not something that most people would choose or ever wish on someone else. Acknowledge to yourself that the stutter is a burden, and it has and will continue to cause you pain. That's just part of the game for us. We can and should minimize its effects through careful management, but it's okay to acknowledge that this is still a burden.

I think it's wise to confront the fact that you did nothing wrong to deserve this burden. Somewhere along the line, for whatever reason, your speech system happened to develop this way, and it's nobody's fault. As far as the current science shows, there is nothing that anyone could have done differently to save you from this lifelong affliction.

It sucks that no matter how hard you work or how carefully you manage it, there will always be the potential to block on any word you say for the rest of your life. That was a very painful lesson when I first learned it.

I experienced a period of rapid personal growth in my early twenties. This newfound maturity and confidence translated to major improvements in my fluency, to the point that I was nearly-perfectly fluent. I thought that I had "beat" my stutter, that with confident action and proper management, my stutter would be a thing of the past.

Then, an obstinate bout of dysfluency set me back. I did some research in hopes of regaining my fluency, and that's when I learned that a stutter can't be eradicated once it persists to adulthood. I had thought that if I worked hard enough and did the "right" things I could free myself of this burden for good, so discovering otherwise was incredibly disheartening. No matter what I did, my stutter would always be a part of me.

It was difficult to come to terms with that reality, but I'm glad that I did; it stops me being upset about my present circumstances or fantasizing about some future miracle cure that will solve the problem for me; my energy only goes towards what I can do about it. Make peace with your reality, grieve for the things you can't have, and move on.

You can work through these feelings in a variety of ways: talk therapy, stuttering support groups, and journaling are all helpful approaches. Professional therapists are experts at working through unpleasant feelings and grief; they can help you work out these feelings in a safe, understanding environment. Similarly, stuttering support groups and talking with others who have had the same thoughts, feelings, and experiences can be deeply validating.

If you prefer to work through these matters on your own, consider writing in a journal. Journaling gives you the freedom to express all of your thoughts and feelings in the comfort of privacy. Sit down with pen and paper or at your computer, and express how you feel about your stutter, how it has affected your life, and what you hope for in the future.

Closing

There is no reason for anyone to suffer through severe dysfluency, restricted agency, or poor mental health; thanks to the research, we know how to manage stuttering so that it is no worse than mild dysfluency. If you follow the guidance of the research literature, you can gain the tools you need to improve your fluency, agency, and well-being.

I know that people can be apprehensive about trying a new "cure" when so many promising treatments have failed in the past; it hurts to feel like you've ended up at the same place where you began despite all your work and sacrifice. I think this is especially true for stuttering, which can be so confusing and unpredictable.

Still, do not let that stop you from committing yourself to the treatments above. These approaches are built on rigorous research and large sample sizes, not a random individual's self-generated theories. They do not promise perfection, but they do offer hope. Have faith that if you put in the time and the effort, you can improve your fluency and your life.

There is reason to be even more optimistic: Mild dysfluency isn't the best possible outcome. Next, we'll set our sights on successful management.

Chapter Nine: Successful Management
Action, Satisfaction, and Near-Fluency

Fall 2016

There's a fantastic burrito shop in downtown Boston called Villa Mexico, run by the mother-daughter team of Bessie and Julie "Momma" King. They are famous for their homemade molé sauce and spicy black salsa. They're also incredibly kind people; I've always loved how Momma King affectionately refers to each customer as "my dear."

I first discovered Villa Mexico when I landed a software job at a nearby tech start-up. Every Wednesday, the company would buy lunch for the software team, and it was up to the six of us to decide where to go. After my first molé burrito, my vote always went to Villa Mexico.

Villa Mexico didn't use the online ordering apps, though, so whenever we chose it for lunch, someone from the team would have to call in the order. Our team lead would always ask "Alright, who wants to make the call?" and, like the stereotypically anti-social software engineers that we were, no one would ever volunteer. We'd all stare at the ground, uncomfortably waiting for someone else to bite the bullet. I thought it was a bit silly that a bunch of grown adults were afraid of a simple phone call, but to be fair, I wasn't volunteering either.

My fluency had regressed in the six months before I joined the company: the job hunt had been stressful and filled with brutal rejections. Once I landed the job, I was overwhelmed by the pace and ambition of start-up life, having spent the previous four years in slow, boring, consequence-free government employment. And since this was my first job as a software engineer, I was very uncertain about my performance; I felt like I was making too many mistakes, not learning fast enough, and generally slowing the team down. In light of all this stress, I was hoping for a respite, for things to get easier – not to add another struggle to my life.

But that scene – no one stepping up to call in lunch – bothered me every time it happened. While I may have had a "better" excuse than my teammates, I couldn't ignore the fact that I was avoiding it, too. It made me feel weak to give in to my fear of stuttering; I hated to think that I was too scared to even try. My frustration at myself and the situation kept building until one week, I volunteered to make the call to Villa Mexico before my boss even asked.

That first call was very stressful. I was worried it would go poorly, so I ducked into a secluded corner of the office where my co-workers wouldn't hear me. I went over the team's orders several times, sketching out a rough script for myself. I centered myself by taking a few slow breaths. I acknowledged to myself that yes, I might stutter badly on the call, and yes, the restaurant may not respond well. The fear was real, but that feeling didn't guarantee that the call would go poorly; I wouldn't know how fluent I would be until I was actually on the phone.

The call, as it turned out, went pretty well. I blocked a little on the initial "Hello," but it's not too unusual for there to be an extra half-second before someone starts speaking on the phone.

After that, my speech came out smoothly. I managed to keep myself calm; I focused on getting the orders right as a way to distract myself from worrying about my fluency.

I felt good about myself afterwards: I hadn't been perfectly fluent, but I had taken on a challenge and done well for myself. It certainly wasn't the trainwreck I had expected.

It was a victory, but I knew I still had room to grow; after all, that was one call to one restaurant. I had overheard dozens of calls that our sales team made from the conference room. They were so confident and smooth on the phone, no matter the time of day or who they were speaking to. I wanted to be like *that*.

So I decided that I would volunteer to call in all of the team's lunch orders from then on. I figured this would give me plenty of opportunities to desensitize myself to the stress and get better at speaking on the phone.

Still, I had doubts about this project of mine. I didn't want my self-improvement to burden others; it wouldn't be fair to make another person deal with me stuttering my way through a phone call just because I thought it would help me. It might be unpleasant to talk with me over the phone, even when I'm fluent; my voice is too deep and nasally for my liking, and my enunciation is generally poor. I decided I'd try to speak slowly and clearly in hopes it would be easier on the listener. At the very least, it was reassuring to know that Bessie and Momma King were very kind people; they would probably never say anything even if I was a burden.

The more of these calls I made, the less stressful they became. They were still the most intense moments of my day, but the feeling gradually shifted from nerve-wracking danger to thrilling challenge. Each time I finished a call, I would pat myself on the back for having taken another step in the right direction. And, as a bonus, there was always the reward of a delicious burrito.

I felt more confident in my speech, but even more than that I loved feeling like I had become a minor hero for taking over the phone calls; it wasn't lost on me that I was the only one on the team with a speech impediment. Plus, I got to form a pleasant relationship with Bessie and Momma

King over several months of calling in orders and going to the shop to pick them up.

One day, as I was picking up an order, Bessie said out of the blue, "You know, you're great on the phone. You're, like, one of my favorite customers." This floored me. I figured that even if I was mostly fluent, my voice would still sound anxious and unpleasant, and my speech wouldn't have the natural, easy flow of fluent speakers. I could not understand for the life of me why Bessie would ever feel that way, so I asked what she meant.

She stopped for a second to think. "You're very... *legible* on the phone. You say it like-" she imitated my cadence and made a clean chopping motion with her hand with each order "One carnitas burrito, extra spicy...' Pause. 'One molé burrito with guacamole...' Pause. 'And one veggie burrito, no onions.' You make it very easy to understand you with the way you speak. Which is helpful, because it can get pretty loud in here."

Like many honest and unexpected compliments, this single remark changed my entire self-concept. I would never have expected anyone to say something positive about my speech, especially the way I speak on the phone. I don't think Bessie said this just to be nice, either; I don't think she knew that I had a stutter or was calling the restaurant as a project to get better on the phone.

When I started calling in these lunch orders, I was just hoping to go from terrible to average; I would have been content with simply not being an obnoxious burden. As it turned out, I had done better than average – I'd even developed some good traits to boot.

This journey didn't just help me with my stutter; it made me more confident in other aspects of my life, too. I became less anxious about my performance as an engineer, I became more social with my co-workers, and I spoke up more often during meetings. I began to feel like I contributed something unique and useful to the team. There were other speaking situations that still scared me, like giving a presentation in front of the entire company, but this experience showed me that if I put my mind to it, I could conquer those challenges as well.

Successful Management

I am not the only stutterer who has gained fluency by taking on speech challenges; I have met others who have become significantly more fluent and confident than when they were younger. Some of the people I've met in support groups and online forums report that while they still have a stutter, they're mostly fluent and much more assertive in when they choose to speak.

There is even a small host of research literature on this "recovery," including studies conducted by Laura Plexico, Christian Kell, Katrin Neumann, Tracy K. Anderson and Susan Felsenfeld. The adult stutterers in these studies had lived with a stutter for their entire lives, but at the time they were interviewed, they were much more fluent and could apply that fluency to situations they would have dreaded or avoided when they were younger.[58,60,61,74,75]

Speech metrics from these studies point to this "recovery" as qualitatively different from what most stutterers experience. Speech therapy improves fluency, but across all the studies discussed so far, almost none of the participants spoke with fewer than 2% stuttered syllables at the end of their program. Additionally, these participants also experienced a temporary drop in speech naturalness.

Recovered stutterers, however, had qualitatively better metrics than the other participants. Recovered participants in these studies spoke with between .8-2% and .2-.8% stuttered syllables, depending on the measurement criteria. What's even more remarkable is that the fluent speakers in one of these studies were measured at .7% stuttered syllables! The recovered participants' speech naturalness was rated only slightly behind that of fluent speakers. The recovered speakers reported more anxiety about speaking situations than fluent speakers, but significantly less anxiety than the therapeutic cohort, either before or after completing speech therapy.

As Laura Plexico pointed out, "recovery" is not the perfect term to describe this phenomenon. While these participants' speech was significantly more fluent and natural than when they were younger, this was not a complete cessation of stuttering, like in childhood recovery. Additionally, these interviewees reported that they needed to actively mind their speech to speak with this level of fluency. For these reasons, Plexico suggested a new term that more accurately describes this phenomenon: "successful management."

I have lived with successful management for over a decade, and while I find that my speech system is more cooperative than when I was younger, I feel that the primary cause of increased fluency comes from an improved ability to monitor my speech and to work through blocks. I sense blocks sooner than I did when I was younger; I can feel a syllable or two ahead that my speech system is "off," and that unless I do something about it, I will probably block.

The adjustments I make while working through blocks are both more subtle and more effective than when I was younger; I almost never experience obstinate blocks anymore. Before successful management, it felt like there was almost nothing I could do to get through a block; my only options were to meet the resistance of a block with more force – which usually only made it more intractable – substitute a different word, or not speak at all. Now, I have the experience and presence of mind to feel where the block "is," untangle it, and apply gentle, guided pressure until I can get through to the other side. These days, managing my speech feels like a yoga teacher gently adjusting a student's posture, rather than a wild animal trying to thrash its way out of a trap.

Because I'm able to get past blocks with only these minor adjustments, my speech usually sounds natural to the average person. While some friends have spent enough time with me to know that I have a stutter, I'm still shocked from time-to-time when I mention my stutter to an acquaintance, and despite my doubts that they're just being polite, they insist they had no idea.

Then again, more than once I've spent several hours listening to a podcast before the guest – often someone relatively famous and successful – has a minor, but undeniable block and I realize that they have a stutter. For instance, I never realized that Shaq – one of the most famous and charismatic people on the planet – had a stutter until I read an interview where he discussed it. Even since learning that he has a stutter, I still find it hard to detect the adjustments he makes to navigate through or around dysfluency.

For me, this improved fluency is closely linked with a stronger sense of agency; I speak more often because I'm more fluent, and I'm more fluent because I speak as soon as I feel the desire to, before doubt and anxiety can creep in.

Recall stuttering's "momentum meter" from Chapter Three. When I was younger and my fear of stuttering kept me from speaking, this momentum meter was almost always in the negative. Now that I've made it a habit of pushing myself out of my comfort zone, I almost always have positive momentum when facing a speaking challenge. I still have bad days and I still shy away from my fair share of challenges, but now, those fluctuations are smaller and easier to recover from.

The habit of tackling challenges head-on actually leads to fewer of these obstacles. Calling a restaurant used to be very stressful, which exacerbated my stutter; but the more often I called Villa Mexico, the easier it became. After a few months, calling a restaurant stopped being such a big deal; I had brought the task inside my comfort zone, so I was less stressed, and fluency came more easily.

I still experience my share of challenging speaking situations; there are still many times when I know I want to speak, but I'm scared about following through on that desire. I try to approach those moments the way a running back faces down a linebacker: My instinct may be to protect myself, but it's actually safest to run directly at the challenge as hard as possible; to meet the danger with strength.

The Neuroscience of Successful Management

Earlier, we explored Christian Kell's research, which compared neurological speech production between stutterers and fluent speakers. He and his team scanned the brains of fluent speakers as the baseline, or "standard" control group. They then scanned a cohort of stutterers before and after intensive speech therapy, and again after the group completed a one-year maintenance program. Comparing these scans showed the differences between fluent speakers and stutterers as well as the changes in stutterers' speech production as they progressed through speech therapy. However, there was a third group in Kell's study: A cohort of those who successfully managed their stutters.[58,61]

Scans showed that those in the successful management cohort shared the same etiological flaws as the therapeutic cohort. However, individuals in the successful management cohort – who did not undergo speech therapy as part of the study – did not have the maladaptations observed in the other stutterers prior to speech therapy. In fact, the beneficial adaptations that only developed for the therapeutic cohort after the maintenance period were already present in the successful management cohort.

When participants in the therapeutic cohort were first scanned, the connections between their auditory and motor cortices were faulty and unreliable. The unreliability of auditory feedback led to an over-reliance on somatosensory feedback for speech planning. Speech therapy restored the auditory-motor connection and brought the auditory-somatosensory balance to a level that matched that of fluent speakers. The participants in the successful management cohort, however, already showed both of these "normal" markers.

The therapeutic cohort members started the study with faulty white matter connections in the LIFG; these connections were only normalized after they had completed the maintenance program. In contrast, participants in the successful management cohort already had healthy white matter connections.

Finally, participants in the therapeutic cohort under-activated the LIFG during emotional and linguistic prosody prior to speech therapy. Speech therapy brought activation up to normal levels for emotional prosody, but it was only after they finished the maintenance program that linguistic prosody was normalized. Here, too, participants in the successful management cohort already had healthy levels of activation for both emotional and linguistic prosody.

These findings suggest that perhaps the people in the successful management cohort are not that different from stutterers who undergo a complete speech therapy program: The successful management cohort had the same etiological flaws observed in the therapeutic cohort and arrived at much the same resolution, but they did so without the aid of speech therapy.

There was, however, one activation pattern that clearly distinguished the successful management cohort not only from members of the therapeutic cohort, but also from the fluent speakers: during speech, the successful management cohort showed activation in their left hemisphere in an area labelled Brodmann's Area 47/12 (L BA 47/12). Neither the therapeutic cohort nor the fluent speakers showed activation in this area at any point in the study. This finding lends further credence to the idea that successful management is a qualitatively different phenomenon.

Kell pointed out that while L BA 47/12 activation clearly and strongly correlates with successful management, it was unclear how it might contribute to the improved fluency of successful management; especially because the speech process normally does not pass through the area surrounding L BA 47/12.

Kell observed that this activation in L BA 47/12 was connected to activation in the superior caudal cerebellum; therefore, L BA 47/12's benefit could somehow be related to the functions of the cerebellum, which contributes to timing, fine motor control, and somatosensory processing. Additionally, since this connection operated entirely outside of the standard speech network, it was doing something novel rather than amplifying or assisting existing processes.

Kell hypothesized that L BA 47/12 could be mediating somatosensory information coming from the cerebellum; this would align with the progression of the auditory-somatosensory balance observed in the therapeutic cohort and even take it one step further. Recall that the therapeutic cohort's improved fluency correlated with a shift in the auditory-somatosensory feedback balance from overly-somatosensory to one that matched fluent speakers. If this hypothesis is correct, L BA 47/12 would tip the auditory-somatosensory balance even further towards auditory feedback by blocking somatosensory information.

Kell's other hypothesis developed as a result of the region in which L BA 47/12 is located: the *orbitofrontal cortex*. The orbitofrontal cortex contributes to planning and decision-making; it takes in information about the present moment, compares it to past experiences, predicts the outcomes of multiple potential actions, and then encourages the actions that it calculates will lead to the best outcomes.

Applied to stuttering and successful management, Kell suggested that the orbitofrontal cortex may be incorporating this highly-useful information from the cerebellum – that is, fine-tuned motor control, somatosensory information, and timing – into the executive control of speech. This additional computation and high-quality information may lead to better awareness of one's speech, allowing stutterers to make conscious and effective interventions in their speech in order to maintain fluency.

I give the most weight to this hypothesis because it aligns with my experience of successful management. Perhaps my improved awareness of my speech comes from the orbitofrontal cortex monitoring the motor components of speech and detecting when something is awry.

Kell's work also offers insight on another major question: whether everyone with a stutter has the potential to reach successful management.

Kell pointed out that while L BA 47/12 activation strongly correlated with successful management, it was unclear *when* this activation pattern began; participants were only scanned years or decades after their self-reported transition to successful management, so it could not be discerned whether this cohort had always activated L BA 47/12 or if it was a neuroplastic adaptation that developed as individuals transitioned into successful management.

If these stutterers had always activated L BA 47/12, then only a certain percentage of stutterers would ever have the potential to achieve successful management. However, if this pattern is a neuroplastic adaptation, then it's more likely that any stutterer could reach successful management.

Based on the existing research, I believe it is most likely that L BA 47/12 activation is a neuroplastic adaptation to behavioral changes, much in the same way that speech therapy can drive neurological adaptations. Experiential research shows that there are replicable patterns of behavior that lead to successful management. These behavioral changes – like greater attention to one's speech – dovetail nicely with the hypothesis that L BA 47/12 contributes to the executive control of speech. To me, it seems the L BA 47/12 activation pattern is the last step in the neurological progression from unguided maladaptation, to normalization through speech therapy, and then to successful management.† This neurological progression mirrors the progressive improvement of fluency in these

---

† To be clear, I don't necessarily think all stutterers experience maladaptations, or require speech therapy to reach mild dysfluency.

stages from moderate-to-severe dysfluency, to mild, to near-natural.

Kell made another interesting discovery, one that shed light on the potential for stutterers to have different severities of etiology. Though a stutterer's dysfluency can vary dramatically, it's likely the case that some stutterers have a "worse" stutter than others. Kell discovered that a participant's fluency status – fluent speaker, stutterer, or successfully-managed stutterer – correlated with the volume of grey matter in their LIFG.

Those in the more-fluent groups generally had more grey matter in the LIFG than their less-fluent peers, though there was overlap between the three cohorts. The fact that participants in the successful management cohort had a higher volume of grey matter than those in the therapeutic cohort may be indicative of a less-severe etiology and could suggest that they may have had an easier path to successful management.

However, I don't believe one should presume the severity of their etiology based on their present fluency. Fluency can vary dramatically throughout one's life, and the worst dysfluency correlates with neurological maladaptations that can reliably be resolved through speech interventions. Additionally, it's worth noting that there was significant overlap between the therapeutic and successful-management cohort.

There is even further reason for optimism: Out of the forty-something individuals in these studies who achieved successful management, none indicated that they had known successful management was even a possibility, much less that they had deliberately aimed for it. Most of the interviewees from Laura Plexico's study were active either in speech pathology or in the stuttering community, yet none reported that they were aware of successful management as a phenomenon. These individuals were simply addressing the immediate problems in their life, unaware that doing so would lead to a significant, lasting improvement in their fluency. If successful management can be achieved by those who did not even know it was possible, then those who aim for it and use the lessons of others are even more likely to reach it.

Furthermore, successful management is built on the foundation of developing healthy coping responses to stuttering. Even if one does not induce neuroplastic change, adopting these changes will almost certainly improve one's quality of life.

To be fair, these studies are informative, but do not guarantee success. The insights that we have about achieving successful management only come from the reports of those who effectively reached successful management. There are no studies that tested – much less proved – the efficacy of a program specifically designed for reaching successful management; it's possible that one could exactly replicate the behaviors and attitudes reported in these studies but not get the same positive results.

However, I believe there is every reason to trust the insights gained from these studies, even though so many things about successful management are still unknown. The two studies on the personal side of successful management – one by Laura Plexico, and the other co-authored by Tracy K. Anderson and Susan Felsenfeld – were conducted independently of each other, yet they reached very similar conclusions. Until future research proves otherwise, I believe we should assume successful management is possible for anyone with a stutter, and that all of us can and should aim for it.

The Transition to Successful Management

Speech therapy is one stepping-stone that helped stutterers achieve successful management, but surprisingly, it is not the most common approach. Of the thirteen participants in Kell's successful-management cohort, only four had ever attended speech therapy, and only one of those four considered it a causal factor in recovery. Even more telling, there was a major gap between when the participants finished therapy and when they made the transition to successful management; this gap was (respectively) five, seven, twenty-six and thirty-eight years. Therefore, while intensive speech therapy can bring severe-to-moderate dysfluency to mild, it does not necessarily continue the journey into successful management.

In her studies on the experiential side of stuttering, Laura Plexico identified two sets of coping mechanisms employed by stutterers to manage life with their speech impediment. The first set of coping mechanisms typified stutterers' experience before successful management, when they were overwhelmed by their stutter and unable to make lasting positive change. During this time, these interviewees were ashamed of their stutter and their inability to control it. They tried to always present themselves as fluent speakers. Anxious about blocking around others, they invested a lot of effort into strategizing about how to handle speaking situations. And when others responded unkindly to their speech, they let it affect them.[76]

The pressure that came with the lack of control over their speech, coupled with the strong internal demands to present as fluent, sometimes became unbearable. When this happened, the interviewees reported that they would resort to avoiding speech altogether; they would stifle their desire to speak and avoid social interactions. These interviewees were conscious that this avoidance offered short-term relief from stuttering yet carried severe long-term negative consequences; avoidance undercut their sense of agency, prevented them from realizing their full potential, and left them socially isolated. Stuck between the threat of dysfluency and the pain of avoidance, these interviewees felt frustrated, helpless, and trapped.

However, the same interviewees who suffered terribly under their stutter were still able to achieve successful management; this change in their lives coincided with a shift in coping strategy from avoidance to approach. Instead of running away from the pain of failure, they took risks in pursuit of success. Instead of viewing their stutter as something over which they had no control, they paid closer attention and investigated how to better manage their fluency. Thrusting themselves into action and looking more closely at their stutter then led to more control over their lives and their speech.[77]

The clearest change came in abandoning avoidance as a primary coping mechanism. Interviewees reported that they understood that avoiding speech for fear of dysfluency did not bring them any closer to a long-term solution; if anything, avoidance guaranteed failure, while taking risks at least carried the possibility of success.

Part of this risk-taking included looking more closely at their speech. Before the transition to successful management, they wanted to think about their speech as little as possible, since doing so usually led to greater self-consciousness and worse dysfluency. As part of this transition, these participants adopted an attitude of curiosity and investigated their speech in order to develop better ways to manage it. With more attention, they learned to make adjustments to be a little more fluent. They took responsibility for their speech, with the attitude that they had the power to influence their fluency for the better. With these changes, fluency became less of a blind gamble and more of a strategic challenge.

Swapping avoidance for approach is simple in concept but difficult in execution; avoidance comes from fear of very real potential of dysfluency and social rejection. It's quite a leap to let go of defensive self-protection and deliberately expose oneself to greater danger. Both the Plexico and Anderson & Felsenfeld studies noted that their participants all showed high levels of motivation and determination.

The studies also laid out the catalysts that triggered the desire for change and the motivations that sustained the participants during this journey. For some, success outside of speech led to increased confidence, which then paved the way for success with stuttering. This confidence may have given the interviewees the desire to "do something" about their speech and the emotional wherewithal to tolerate the inevitable setbacks that come with self-improvement. They also learned to see themselves beyond their stutter, as a complete human being, so that their self-concept was no longer dominated by their speech impediment. They also came to recognize that everyone has their struggles in life, that no one really skates through life easily; stuttering just happens to be a problem they had to face.

Of Kell's thirteen successful management participants, four attributed their improvement to professional success or milestones like graduating school. Three attributed it to self-development practices like self-observation, therapy and self-help, or "natural therapy."

Some interviewees credited their success to the support of others: speech therapists, mentors, friends, family, or loved ones. By providing freedom from judgment, these trusted individuals helped the interviewees feel safe from the constant danger of stuttering. Additionally, these people believed in the interviewees' potential to succeed and encouraged their efforts.

One gentleman described how the classic "fake it til you make it" strategy drove his journey to successful management: After he became a police officer, he needed to exude confidence and assertiveness to do his job properly. Initially, this confidence was just an act that he would put on; however, *pretending* to be confident and self-assured for long enough led him to genuinely *feeling* confident and self-assured.

Others confronted their speech first, and this action led to improved fluency and confidence. This is perhaps a more difficult approach, since one has to take risks without the security of a safe retreat.

For some, negative experiences were the catalyst; one interviewee reported that a stern talking-to from a high school teacher made her mad enough to confront the problem of her stutter. With so much pent-up frustration at dysfluency and self-imposed limitations – and nothing left to lose – these participants threw themselves into the speaking situations they had been avoiding. They didn't necessarily have much knowledge about stuttering or a plan for how to improve their fluency, they simply figured it out along the way.

Another interviewee credited his recovery to speech therapy in combination with social support and personal action. For the first thirty years of his life, he was severely distressed and hemmed in by his stutter. On the advice of his then-girlfriend, he enrolled in speech therapy, where he learned for the first time that it was possible to mitigate his dysfluency. Developing the power to work through blocks gave him a sense of agency and showed him that he could push back on his stutter. He displayed his motivation and commitment in continuing to practice therapeutic techniques on his own for a year after therapy.

Others didn't have to motivate themselves into action; they were thrown into the deep end, and to their own surprise, learned that they could swim. One shared that, upon joining the military, he was assigned to deliver aptitude tests. This meant standing in front of a classroom of fresh-faced recruits, giving instructions and answering questions. At first, this was so terrifying that he would numb himself with pills just to get by. But with time and experience, he learned to navigate the situation. As the stress decreased, he became more confident and pushed himself to take on more challenges like making eye contact with recruits while speaking. This deep immersion led to a rapid decrease in his stuttering in only six months; a relatively fast transformation considering that most interviewees reported that their transition took place over six-to-twelve months.

Regardless of the motivation or circumstances, these interviewees show that it's necessary to directly confront one's stuttering in order to reach successful management. These interviewees also offer insight into specific tactics that are essential to this journey.

Redefining "Failure"

If one's goal is successful management, a reasonable, understandable way to measure progress would be one's fluency; but these interviews suggest that this is not the best approach. Interviewees from these studies reported that when they were younger and more dysfluent, they judged their success in a particular situation by how *fluent* they were. This mindset can be unhelpful, though, because by this criteria, stuttering was always equated with failure. If one thinks they will be dysfluent – and thus fail – they will also be more likely to avoid a speaking situation. Additionally, the standard of perfection is an impossible pressure to live up to, even under successful management; if a stutter persists into adulthood, there will always be the potential to block.

Instead, these interviewees redefined failure to mean *failure to try*. What came to matter most was whether they took the initiative to speak, not necessarily how fluent they were when they spoke. This mindset is helpful because it incentivizes action and risk-taking, which are two key drivers of successful management. If you aim high but come up short, then at least you know that you had the courage to try; nothing ventured, nothing gained. If you fail to act, however, you will be stuck wondering "What if?"

These studies underscore the idea that you don't need to wait for improved fluency to increase your agency; in fact, causation usually works in the other direction. To this point, participants in the Menzies study on cognitive-behavioral therapy were able to complete more items on their challenge tasklist even with zero improvements to their fluency.

Losses and rough days are inevitable on this journey. Keep in mind that not all bravery is rewarded in the short-term; sometimes, taking bigger risks will only lead to bigger losses. That's why, in addition to bravery, you need *resilience*.

Resilience

While the achievements of these interviewees are encouraging, it's important to remember that success rarely comes without struggles and setbacks. In my experience, successful management is not a permanent achievement; it's not like you cross a clear threshold and then have a lifetime of easier fluency ahead of you. It may be possible to regress out of successful management. I know that, at times, I have lost that forward-leaning positive momentum; I've felt my comfort zone shrink and my ability to expand it become weakened.

At age twenty-four, I had gotten a grip on my fluency and was becoming more confident in my life and my speech. Had I known about it at the time, I would have considered myself to have reached successful management; I probably would have bet money that I had L BA 47/12 activation, the works. Then, I went to boot camp.

The stress of boot camp shook my fluency and undermined my ability to speak in spite of fear. I fell a long way down into avoidance and negative momentum before I was able to stop the slide. I had to build positive momentum and my sense of agency bit by bit from the ground up. I had to push myself to do things that used to be easy.

Just as we should not expect fluency every time we speak, we should not always expect bravery from ourselves, either. Sometimes, we don't have the emotional bandwidth to do "the right thing." We all experience times where we are too stressed or tired to take a risk, or we simply won't want to deal with the stutter in that moment.

Resilience means bouncing back after defeats and staying focused on the bigger picture. Temporary discouragement is natural, but you need to be able to move on and get the next one. Keep that larger positive momentum rolling, don't let individual losses knock you too far off your game. No matter how bad things may feel at a given moment, the smallest victory can turn the tide.

Speech Management

Participants in these studies reported several speech habits that they considered crucial to managing their fluency. While the increased attention to speech required by these habits may be uncomfortable at first, the stress and discomfort fades away with time, leaving only the calm presence of mind that is needed to make fine-tuned adjustments to speech. Whereas the fluency-shaping techniques used in speech therapy always require attention and effort, these changes can eventually become effortless, unconscious habits.

We stutterers tend to feel like we need to start speaking as soon as it is our "turn"; we have our finger on the trigger, anxiously itching to squeeze it the millisecond someone answers our phone call. This impulse to speak right away only creates tension, which may further compound anxiety. Instead of racing ahead, relax that tension and allow yourself a half-second before you speak. Fluent speakers often take a moment to collect their thoughts before they start speaking; there's nothing wrong with doing the same. In general, practice being relaxed in the moments leading up to speaking; calm confidence leads to better fluency than impatient anxiety.

In a similar vein, practice speaking a little more slowly than you otherwise would. Dysfluency aside, stutterers generally speak at a faster rate than fluent speakers. This difference can be even greater if you're trying to rush through speech before dysfluency strikes. Speaking more slowly brings a host of benefits. It provides more time to notice and maneuver around blocks before they become too entrenched. Think of it like driving: you're better able to spot and avoid potholes when you slow down. Speaking at a slow, controlled pace also reduces the odds that you meet the resistance of a block by pushing against it with brute force. Or, if the block is too difficult to work through, this strategy affords the presence of mind to stop and start over, which will likely be more effective than continuing to push against it.

Stutterers also have a peculiar habit of running out of breath when we speak. This happens when we start speaking on a shallow breath or fail to refill our lungs while we're speaking. Sometimes, when we're down to our last few molecules of oxygen, we'll try to push the words out by squeezing harder on our diaphragm and speech muscles; this is not effective for fluency, nor is it a pleasant sensation.

It's much more effective – and less stressful – to speak with proper breath support. It's so obvious that it seems silly to think about it, but make sure to breathe before you start speaking. Then, as you're speaking, pay attention to how much breath you have left. When you feel like you're running low, pause for a second to breathe, and then carry on. At first, these maintenance breaths may come at unnatural times; that's fine. With practice, it becomes easier to foresee when you will run out of breath, and you can place those maintenance breaths at more natural times. Eventually, you will always speak with proper breath support without even paying attention to it.

A primary component of successful management's improved fluency is having a better understanding of one's speech and fluency. Interviewees in the studies reported that this awareness came through speech practices that they devised themselves as part of their transition.

One interviewee would read aloud from a dictionary while standing in front of a mirror. Another enrolled in Toastmasters, a group where members practice public speaking in front of each other. I found benefit by reading aloud from the prose of Ralph Waldo Emerson; President Joe Biden has said that he would read aloud from Emerson's poetry. Demosthenes, a politician in Ancient Greece, would practice oratory with pebbles in his mouth while standing on a cliff in front of a roaring ocean.

Developing your own practice will give you more exposure to the subtleties of managing your speech and a safe place to practice working through blocks. Whatever practice you end up doing, the most important thing is that it works for you and that you can stick to it.

A Cure for Stuttering?

In many ways, it's unfortunate that no amount of proper management will eradicate the stutter; that the benefits "only" top out at successful management. It would be nice if, having done all the work to reach successful management, my speech impediment would go away for good, like I once thought it did when I first started becoming more fluent. Or, if I only blocked when I committed some kind of "fault." It would be nice if I could keep all the positive traits I developed because of my stutter and slough off stuttering for good, but that just doesn't seem to be the way it works.

The holy grail of stuttering research would be a cure for stuttering; to completely remove the proclivity to block, whether through brain surgery, a pill, or some other intervention. Could science develop this "cure" for stuttering? It's entirely possible, but I'm not optimistic.

The brain is a complex organ that we do not fully understand, nor does it seem like the etiology of stuttering is limited to only a few neurological processes, or even a few parts of the brain. The more areas of the brain that need to be changed, the harder it becomes to fix the problem, and the greater the risk of side effects. And while much progress has been made in the past twenty years in understanding the etiology of stuttering and how stutterers' brains differ from those of fluent speakers, it's also likely that we do not yet have the complete picture. So I am very skeptical that an intervention will be developed in my lifetime that can fix the root causes of stuttering without somehow mucking up something else.

If an operation or treatment was developed, I wouldn't be one of the early adopters. My stutter is still a burden in my life, and I would be incredibly grateful if it disappeared tomorrow – the day my stutter disappeared would be one of the best days of my life – but my stutter is not such an intractable problem that I would risk tampering with my brain. It's unfortunate that my brain produces stuttered speech, but it could be a lot worse.

I am, however, much more optimistic about "curing" stuttering in children. Natural recovery already exists in children, so – unlike adult recovery – it wouldn't require creating a completely novel phenomenon.

Research by Ho Ming Chow and Soo-Eun Chang has given us our first look at *how* children's brains change as they recover from stuttering, though we still know almost nothing about *why* those children recover and others don't.

If future research can discover what causes certain children to recover, we could learn how to induce recovery in children whose stutter would otherwise persist. If this were to happen, we could eradicate stuttering from future generations, which would be an incredible achievement.

I may be overly pessimistic in my predictions. Scientific breakthroughs are impossible to predict, and the pace of research may increase beyond anything I expected. I would never rule out the possibility that a safe and effective cure for adults could be developed in the near future. That said, partly for my own mental health, partly because I think it is a more "effective" belief, I shade towards pessimism.

There is risk in hoping for an external resolution to your stutter, rather than learning to mitigate it yourself. If you expect a cure in the future, you may lose the motivation to do the work that has been demonstrated to improve fluency. However, if you put in the effort because you do not expect a cure, but then your stutter is resolved, you lose nothing.

The Joy of Successful Management

Successful management of stuttering is characterized by an **optimistic and positive interpretation of life**. In spite of the fact that self-management of stuttering continues, the possibility of stuttering is no longer a major theme. There is a sense of appreciation for what has been accomplished. Although speakers are considerably more fluent than in the past, more dominant themes indicate that life choices are no longer restricted by anxiety or fear associated with stuttering or the possibility of stuttering. **There is an obvious sense of freedom to act and speak on one's own behalf.**

-Laura Plexico (emphasis added)

When you're living in the deep darkness of stuttering, it may seem like you will never be able to truly live – that you will never be able to express yourself, to socialize, to feel comfortable. But we are fortunate that there is hope; it is possible to live a full life despite this speech impediment – to say what you want to say, when you want to say it.

Even better, we know how to get all the way from severe dysfluency and limitation to successful management. There is no reason to believe that the freedom and agency of successful management is impossible for anyone with a stutter, regardless of their current state.

Successful management is the best possible outcome as far as we know, but it demands that you earn it. The journey to greater fluency and agency may be difficult.

It may even be the hardest thing you've ever done. But you are the only person who can do the work needed to reach your goals, and you are the only person who knows how to motivate yourself into action.

When the journey gets difficult, I encourage you to think of what Laura Plexico wrote above.

The past few chapters have been about the work of climbing up the mountain; the toil and suffering necessary to get from dysfluency and despair to fluency and agency. The journey isn't painless, but when you reach the summit, you can sit down, relax, and enjoy the view.

Chapter Ten: From Here
Life Beyond Stuttering

Fall 2018

    I landed a new tech job in late summer of 2018. The company was fairly large, so new hires like myself went through quite a few onboarding sessions to get up to speed. Three months into my tenure, I was down to my last training, a one-hour session titled "Living the Company Values." I wasn't thrilled about it.

    I resented how so many events at these modern tech companies come with a sense of forced fun, this unspoken feeling of "Wow, aren't we all such great friends here?" For that reason, it had crossed my mind to skip this "company values" session, but the company had treated me well so far and the earlier technical trainings had been very insightful; I figured there was no harm in sitting through one more session.

    I walk into a large conference room and see one hundred other recent hires, all seated facing the front of the room; it seems like this session will be one long lecture. I take a seat and prepare to zone out for the next hour. *Well, if this is how the company wants to spend its money*, I think.

    The training leader calls in everyone's attention and gives us a short spiel about the company values. Then, to my surprise, he says that we're going to split into discussion groups. He counts us off and sends each group to one of the ten poster boards hung up around the room.

    Once there, he gives us our next set of instructions. "You are all standing in front of one of the ten company values. Your task, as a group, is to share examples that you have seen of the company values in action, and then write them down on your poster."

Our poster says "We are confident, but humble."

Our group starts off with an uncertain, standoff-ish vibe, but as we go around sharing stories, we become more comfortable with each other.

One woman offers "I think the 'open office' setup shows that everyone is valued equally, that no one is 'too important.' I started here three weeks ago and the CEO literally sits two desks over from me. He doesn't hide in a private office in the corner of the building; he does the 'open office' thing like everyone else. And that means every other manager down the line has to be accessible, too."

"Okay, time's up!" yells the trainer from the center of the room. I figure we'll rotate to the next poster over and repeat the process. I'm surprised when the trainer then says "Now let's go around the room and have each group present their company value and one or two items from their list. So everyone, nominate someone from your group to be the spokesperson."

Suddenly, our group gets closed off again; arms fold over chests and eyes fall to the ground. It seems like no one from our group wants to speak in front of a hundred strangers. Except for me, that is – I don't mind at all.

At this point in my life, I'm fairly comfortable with public speaking. It used to terrify me, but I had done it enough times by this point that I actually feel quite confident. Presenting for our group would still be a challenge, but I knew I could manage myself and my speech in spite of the pressure.

But I don't volunteer right away; I wait a few extra seconds to allow someone else the opportunity to step up. I don't have anything to prove to myself anymore when it comes to public speaking, but maybe someone else in the group is where I was only a little while ago, eager to conquer the challenge. Odds are, though, no one else will step up.

After a beat of silence, I put my hand up. "I can do it. I don't mind." The tension dissipates and I feel a stab of pride; I, the one person in the group with a stutter, just bailed out the fluent speakers.

I shift into preparation mode. I know from experience that I'm terrible at speaking off the top of my head; I tend to lose my train of thought or spiral off on a rambling tangent. Having a rough idea of what to say also keeps me grounded during the initial rush that comes with public speaking.

I look over the team's stories on our poster. I thought it was really interesting that the CEO of a billion-dollar company sits ten feet away from a recent hire, so I sketch out a loose script for myself based on that story. I also grab one of the group's markers so I can fiddle with something in my hands.

The trainer picks up again. "Does each group have a spokesperson?" He looks around the room and gets affirmative nods in response.

I figure he's going to pick a group to go first. I am surprised, yet again, when he asks "Okay, who'd like to go first?" I look around at the other groups; no hands go up.

Another wave of calm confidence washes over me. It's the same situation all over again. I wait to see if someone else will volunteer.

I can feel the tension rise as the seconds tick by. I figure the trainer doesn't want to force one of the groups to go first. Nor do I think anyone wants to be forced into it, either.

I raise my hand again. The trainer notices and gestures my way. "Great! We'll start with this group here. Tell us what your company value was, and share a story or two."

I feel the weight of a hundred pairs of eyes falling on me. It's a little overwhelming, but practice has helped me master the adrenaline rush, to enjoy the thrill. I'm in control, after all; I chose this.

As I speak, I look back and forth from our poster to various people in the crowd. I never hold eye contact for more than a second or two; that extra stimulation could trip up my fluency or my train of thought.

"Our value was 'We are confident, but humble.' One of the people in our group-"

"Can't hear you!" comes a shout from across the room.

The sudden interruption stops me in my tracks. I'm a little irritated; maybe this guy couldn't hear me very well, but he definitely could have been more polite about it. Still, he has a point; he's thirty yards away, and the noise from the cafeteria next door is bleeding into our room.

I exhale sharply through my nose and mentally reset. I start again, this time raising my voice.

"Our group's value was 'We are confident, but humble.' One of the people in our group-"

"Still can't hear you!" *Same freaking guy.*

Now I'm more than a little irritated, but I stay within myself; I can't afford to lose my composure because it would ruin my fluency, and I want to do a good job of this.

Okay, I think to myself. *You want loud? I can do loud.* At the time, I was only a few years removed from boot camp, where I had to yell at the top of my lungs every time I spoke for eight weeks. I know I can be loud enough for my friend in the corner to hear me just fine.

I inhale through my nose and project my voice loud and deep: "OUR GROUP'S VALUE WAS-"

I'm so loud that I can see the trainer – only ten yards away – blink his eyes and pull his head back in shock.

"WE ARE CONFIDENT BUT HUMBLE.' ONE OF OUR GROUP MEMBERS SITS ONLY A FEW DESKS AWAY FROM THE CEO."

I could probably dial it back, lower my voice a few decibels, but I keep it up just to prove a point. Plus, the sheer absurdity of being this loud takes the edge off my nerves.

"SHE WAS REALLY IMPRESSED THAT HE STILL WORKS AT AN OPEN OFFICE DESK LIKE THE REST OF US, NOT BEHIND A DOOR IN A CORNER OFFICE. THAT SETS AN EXAMPLE FOR ALL THE OTHER MANAGERS TO FOLLOW."

I smile and nod politely to the trainer to let him know I'm done.

"Well, uh, thank you for that," he says. "Now let's go around the rest of the room, starting with this group to the left."

As we go around the room, the rest of the groups present their stories – without further interruptions from my friend in the corner.

When I think back on this memory, I'm still proud of myself. It wasn't just that I had spoken well that day, but that I had come so far from when I was younger. Ten years earlier, I would have never volunteered to speak for the group, or to present first; the prospect of speaking in front of a hundred strangers would have been terrifying.

But I had slowly improved my confidence and public speaking ability by taking on small challenges. I did public speaking so many times when I was afraid that it began to scare me less, and I learned to speak in spite of my fear. It wasn't just one victory; it made it clear that all those small moments of bravery had paid off, too.

I didn't succeed because my stutter had gone away; I succeeded because I had become stronger than it.

"Who would you be if you never had a stutter?"

I think everyone with a stutter wonders how their life would be different if they never had a stutter. The most common response I've seen in online forums is something like "If not for the stutter, I would be incredibly social and confident. I would make tons of friends and speak my mind without any worries." I understand why someone with a stutter would feel this way, but personally, I don't think it's realistic or productive.

Severe dysfluency causes so much stress and anxiety that other, smaller problems are blocked out by the stutter. It may seem like all of your social interactions would go smoothly if you didn't have a stutter, but fluent speakers still have plenty of awkward and unpleasant social interactions. Even if you don't have to worry whether your words will come out, you still have to worry that you will choose the *right words* to say. So I think it's important not to overestimate the effect your stutter has on your social interactions, or to have an idealized version of what life is like as a fluent speaker.

Up until you experience successful management, it's likely that the stutter will be a huge factor in your life, whether that's because you're suffering under the weight of it, or you're doing the hard work to improve your fluency. During that time, it may seem like the stutter will be in the foreground of your mind for the rest of your life; but that probably won't be the case. In my experience, once you reach the less-intense period of maintenance, you experience less suffering and with less effort than ever before; the stutter won't disappear from your life, but it does fade into the background.

Nor would I say that my stutter has only had a negative effect on me and my life so far. True, having a stutter has caused suffering I would not have experienced if I was a fluent speaker, but at the same time, battling this disorder has made me stronger in ways I maybe otherwise would not be.

Negative Incentive, Positive Outcome

I have a bad habit of binge-eating peanut M&M's; I can easily eat a pound of them in a single sitting. I know it's not healthy, and I know I shouldn't do it, but I still do it because the negative effects aren't painful enough. My stomach feels funny for an hour or two, and I probably gain some weight that I don't really notice. But that's not enough to outweigh the pleasurable dopamine rush that I get from eating chocolate and sugar, so my bad habit continues.

If I was diabetic, though, I bet I'd kick the habit pretty quickly. If that was the case, eating a pound of chocolate could send me into diabetic coma. That danger would be a powerful *negative incentive*† to exert more self-control over my diet. In the same way, a stutter is a *negative incentive* that can lead to beneficial outcomes.

We know that a variety of factors can make a stutter worse in both the short- and long-term: stress, anxiety, nerves, lack of confidence, avoidance. While it is

---

† A negative incentive encourages certain behaviors through punishment, or the threat thereof: I know my grandma will slap my hand if I reach for a cookie before dinner, so I keep my hands to myself.

unfortunate that a stutter punishes you for states that are already unpleasant and unhelpful, it also means you can use your stutter as a negative incentive to avoid those states. The added visceral unpleasantness of blocking has motivated me to take better care of myself. For me, the clearest result has been developing a mindfulness practice.

When I was younger, I struggled with ADD, anxiety, and maintaining my composure under stress. While they all negatively affected my quality of life, I felt the pain most sharply in my speech. Considering how badly anxiety exacerbated my stutter, I recognized that developing self-management would greatly improve my fluency. Motivated by the desire to reduce my stuttering, I started mindful meditation when I was twenty-five years old.

People generally know that regular meditation can lead to a host of benefits, yet they still struggle to stick with the practice past the first few weeks. That's because the discomfort that sometimes comes with meditation is immediate and obvious, but the benefits are subtle and take time. For me, even slight improvements in my ability to maintain my composure led to noticeably better fluency. Having a stutter provided that extra incentive I needed to stick to the practice long enough to make it a regular part of my life.

I still have ADD, I still experience high levels of anxiety, and I still experience lots of stimulation during stressful moments, but mindfulness allows me to separate those sensations from how I feel and act. This makes me more resilient in the face of stress, and as an added bonus, I'm able to keep myself in better baseline states. These changes were developed primarily because of my stutter, and I still feel them most clearly in my speech, but they have benefited me in other areas of life as well.

I have friends who are liable to say unkind and unhelpful things when stressed or frustrated – things that would have been better left unsaid, if they had been able to stop themselves. I have been in those same situations, feeling that same intense urge to vent my frustration, but mindfulness helped me stay within myself. My stutter stopped me from speaking once again, but this time in a helpful way.

This mindfulness doesn't only mitigate negatives; it increases positives, too. Mindfulness helps with detachment from unpleasant sensations while also allowing you to experience and enjoy even more of the pleasant. I'm a very excitable person, and when I was younger, I would sometimes get so happy or excited that I would lose my composure and stutter more. Now, I'm actually able to experience that joy to a deeper level – and stay fluent – in those moments thanks to my mindfulness practice.

Mindfulness has also made me braver. I believe people often fear saying kind things to other people because giving an honest compliment makes you vulnerable. You can pour your heart out in a generous way only to get rejected with a funny look – or worse. I know that I've withheld compliments for fear of embarrassing myself before, but with the greater equanimity that's come from mindfulness, I say more kind things that otherwise may have been left unspoken.

My stutter has also broadened my personality; by default, I tend to be cautious and strategic, but my stutter has taught me to be courageous. I have ran away from the threat of blocking enough times to know that I am safest by throwing myself forward, even when I'm scared, even when I don't know what will come of it. I've learned that it's better to die trying than to feel regret for the rest of my life.

Seeing Hell From Heaven

When my life first started to improve, I didn't want to look back on the suffering I had been through. The wounds were still too fresh, and I worried that looking back on the way I used to live would drag me right back into that existence. If I could have erased those memories of suffering from my mind, I would have.

With time I was able to accept that my newfound fluency and agency were secure, and that if I did regress, I knew how to climb back up again.

Comparing my life to what it used to be, I feel grateful for what I have today, and – like Laura Plexico wrote – I feel a sense of accomplishment for what I've achieved. When I think about simple tasks that used to terrify me – like phone calls – I'm proud to say that I now do those things routinely. Contrasting my old self with my current self is no longer scary; it has become a source of confidence.

In my experience, when someone is confident, others tend to assume that person has always been that way. They think the world has always flung its doors open for these people, and that they can boldly venture forth only because they have never tasted failure or deep suffering.

I believe the opposite is true. Deep, unshakeable confidence doesn't come from never having lost: it comes from failing terribly, getting back to your feet, and then succeeding. True confidence comes from knowing that you can take risks because no matter how badly you fail, you know you will get up, dust yourself off, and keep striving.

I learned this because of my stutter. The failure and suffering I've experienced has not left me scarred, hobbled, or afraid; it has only made me stronger. Nothing can throw me back into the deep pit of suffering and hopelessness that used to be my daily reality.

Even if I lost everything I have today, I know I would be alright: I dug myself out once before, I can do it again.

From Here

I will likely stutter for the rest of my life. I doubt that I will ever be able to speak with complete confidence that the words will actually come out. I may even see this affliction eradicated in future generations, while I am "grandfathered in" with my stutter. In the one life I was given, I had to live with a stutter.

I'm comfortable with that reality; that's just how life turned out for me. I consider myself fortunate in that there are much worse afflictions, and there are conditions that cannot be mitigated no matter how hard one works.

As difficult as it has been to combat my stutter, I'm grateful for the journey. It was incredibly painful at times, but I know that the worst is behind me. I wouldn't say that I would have had a *better* life if I never had my stutter, only that I would have a *different* one.

From here, I'll keep investing time and effort into my speech. In the short-term, I'll devote a small percentage of my brainpower to monitoring my speech, like a background process on a computer. I'll watch my speech over the longer-term and set aside time to read aloud if my fluency starts to drop too much. These are just simple things I have to do to keep myself on the right track; a matter of discipline like staying on top of my dietary habits and exercise routine.

There will be lots of tiny victories because of my stutter – times when I push past my fear of blocking and say exactly what I want to. There will be times when I get through a potentially-dangerous block. Or someone will be impressed by a presentation I gave, when that person didn't even know that I have a stutter.

And there will be bad days, too. I will block. I will substitute words. I'll stay silent for fear of blocking. And some people will respond unkindly to my speech.

But hey, I'll be fine. I've been through worse.

Acknowledgments

My first and foremost thanks must go to my editor, Steffannie Alter. In most author-editor partnerships, the editor receives the author's final draft, makes some alterations, and then the book is published. Not so in my case. Mrs. Alter was an active collaborator who provided insightful, invaluable feedback throughout the entire writing process; be that sifting through the tangled mess of early drafts, to sharpening and refining final drafts. There were many times when I was stuck on a particularly trying section, knowing it was flawed but clueless as how to fix it, when I calmed myself with the refrain "Steffannie will know what to do about this." In all honestly, no obstacle could have stopped me from finishing this book save for losing the contribution of Mrs. Alter.

I would like to thank Andrew Etchell for providing both technical feedback and support through this process. I originally reached out to Andrew to ask questions about his work, but his interest and support for the project turned into greatly-appreciated regular correspondence.

I would like to thank Randy Panzarino for his support as well as providing technical feedback about the effects of stuttering on mental health.

I would like to thank Marie-Christine Franken. When I reached out to her about long-term results for the RESTART study, she invited me to attend the 2022 International Fluency Association conference, which was a tremendous experience and learning opportunity. Dr. Franken generously took time to discuss her work one-on-one with me and has been incredibly supportive of the project. I would also like to thank Caroline de Sonneville, who connected me with Dr. Franken.

I would like to thank the researchers and academics who took some of their time to answer questions and provide expert technical feedback: Shanqing Cai, Soo-Eun Chang, Christian Kell, Katrin Neumann, Dillon Pruett, Shahriar Sheikh-Bahaei, and Evan Usler. Any errors that remain are solely my responsibility.

I would like to thank the researchers and academics who provided a random inquirer like myself with journal papers that were locked behind expensive paywalls: Ashley Craig, Rahsan Kemerdere, Yoshikazu Kikuchi, and Akira Toyomura (who also sent the Daiki Miyashiro study).

This project would not have been possible without Google Scholar. That tool allowed me – an independent, amateur non-academic – to traverse the vast research literature on stuttering. In a similar vein, I owe a great debt to websites that remove barriers in the way of science.

I would like to thank my childhood friend Jake Tanenbaum for expanding the academic scope of this book from one study to the two-hundred-odd studies I ended up reading. It was Jake that suggested I use Google Scholar to read all the papers cited in Kell 2009, and the papers that cited Kell 2009. This one insight led to a three-month wiki-walk that forever altered how I understand stuttering.

I would like to thank my friend Mike Pepi for convincing me to self-publish this book.

I owe a great debt to the work of Joseph Henrich (*The Secret of Our Success*, *The WEIRDest People in the World*) and Charles Murray (*Human Diversity*) for providing examples of how academic research could be translated into pleasing, readable prose. I also owe a debt to Robert Caro (*The Power Broker*) for his example of how to take a lone stand against a large, established institution.

I thank Robert Bertsche for his invaluable legal advice.

I would like to thank the friends whose interest and support has helped sustain me through these five long years: Blanca, "Bookee," Chris and Rachel, Margot and Michael, Patrick and Julia, Ravi, Rick, Sivan, Sybille, the team at Braven, and everyone at Church Community Builder, especially the Luna team.

I owe a special debt to the family at Church Community Builder, particularly Erik Cramer, who, by allowing me to work less than forty hours per week in December 2019, gave me the time to spend more than two or three sessions a week on this book, and the mental space to think to google "What causes stuttering?" during a writing session in January 2020.

I would like thank the Cambridge Public Library and Minuteman Library Network for enabling me to read so broadly and frequently, and the Harvard Book Store Author Series for exposing me to so many great writers.

I owe a special thanks to everyone in my life who has tolerated my flaws with grace and patience, seen more in me than I saw in myself, or believed in the best of what I was trying to do.

If you enjoyed the book and would like to support it, please consider leaving a review online. All reviews will be read by the author.

References

1. Yairi, Ehud, and Nicoline Ambrose. "Epidemiology of stuttering: 21st century advances." *Journal of fluency disorders* 38.2 (2013): 66-87.

2. Whitebread, G. (2014). A review of stuttering in signed languages. In D. Quinto-Pozos (Ed.), *Multilingual aspects of signed language communication and disorder* (pp. 143-161). Bristol, UK: Multilingual Matters.

3. Cripps, Jody H. "Stuttering-Like Behaviors in American Sign Language Jody H. Cripps Mark W. Pellowski Ellen Fromm."

4. Snyder, Greg. "The Existence of Stuttering in Sign Language and other Forms of Expressive Communication: Sufficient Cause for the Emergence of."

5. See list of articles cited in the second paragraph of Guntupalli 2006 (citation #6).

6. Guntupalli, Vijaya K., et al. "Psychophysiological responses of adults who do not stutter while listening to stuttering." *International journal of psychophysiology* 62.1 (2006): 1-8.

7. Guntupalli, Vijaya K., et al. "Emotional and physiological responses of fluent listeners while watching the speech of adults who stutter." *International Journal of Language & Communication Disorders* 42.2 (2007): 113-129.

8. Blood, Gordon W., and Ingrid M. Blood. "Bullying in adolescents who stutter: Communicative competence and self-esteem." *Contemporary Issues in Communication Science and Disorders* 31. Spring (2004): 69-79.

9. American Psychiatric Association. (2013). *Diagnostic and statistical manual of mental disorders* (5th ed.). https://doi.org/10.1176/appi.books.9780890425596

10. Blumgart, Elaine, Yvonne Tran, and Ashley Craig. "Social anxiety disorder in adults who stutter." *Depression and anxiety* 27.7 (2010): 687-692.

11. Tran, Yvonne, Elaine Blumgart, and Ashley Craig. "Subjective distress associated with chronic stuttering." *Journal of fluency disorders* 36.1 (2011): 17-26.

12. Iverach, Lisa, et al. "Prevalence of anxiety disorders among adults seeking speech therapy for stuttering." *Journal of anxiety disorders* 23.7 (2009): 928-934.

13. Craig, Ashley, Elaine Blumgart, and Yvonne Tran. "The impact of stuttering on the quality of life in adults who stutter." *Journal of fluency disorders* 34.2 (2009): 61-71.

14. Corcoran, Joseph A., and Moira Stewart. "Stories of stuttering: A qualitative analysis of interview narratives." *Journal of Fluency Disorders* 23.4 (1998): 247-264.

15. Plexico, Laura W., Walter H. Manning, and Heidi Levitt. "Coping responses by adults who stutter: Part I. Protecting the self and others." *Journal of fluency disorders* 34.2 (2009): 87-107.

16. Manning, Walter, and J. Gayle Beck. "Personality dysfunction in adults who stutter: Another look." *Journal of Fluency Disorders* 38.2 (2013): 184-192.

17. Panzarino, Randy W. "Psychological Distress and Affective, Behavioral and Cognitive Experiences of Stuttering." (2021).

18. Polikowsky, Hannah G., et al. "Population-based genetic effects for developmental stuttering." *Human Genetics and Genomics Advances* 3.1 (2022): 100073.

19. Frigerio-Domingues, Carlos, and Dennis Drayna. "Genetic contributions to stuttering: the current evidence." *Molecular genetics & genomic medicine* 5.2 (2017): 95-102.

20. Barnes, Terra D., et al. "A mutation associated with stuttering alters mouse pup ultrasonic vocalizations." *Current Biology* 26.8 (2016): 1009-1018.

21. Han, Tae-Un, et al. "Human GNPTAB stuttering mutations engineered into mice cause vocalization deficits and astrocyte pathology in the corpus callosum." *Proceedings of the National Academy of Sciences* 116.35 (2019): 17515-17524.

22. Personal correspondence with Dr. Sheikh-Bahaei.

23. Chow, Ho Ming, and Soo-Eun Chang. "White matter developmental trajectories associated with persistence and recovery of childhood stuttering." *Human brain mapping* 38.7 (2017): 3345-3359.

24. Usler, Evan, and Christine Weber-Fox. "Neurodevelopment for syntactic processing distinguishes childhood stuttering recovery versus persistence." *Journal of neurodevelopmental disorders* 7 (2015): 1-22.

25. Usler, Evan, Anne Smith, and Christine Weber. "A lag in speech motor coordination during sentence production is associated with stuttering persistence in young children." *Journal of Speech, Language, and Hearing Research* 60.1 (2017): 51-61.

26. Bohland, Jason W., Daniel Bullock, and Frank H. Guenther. "Neural representations and mechanisms for the performance of simple speech sequences." *Journal of cognitive neuroscience* 22.7 (2010): 1504-1529.

27. Yairi, Ehud, and Nicoline Grinager Ambrose. "Early childhood stuttering I: Persistency and recovery rates." *Journal of Speech, Language, and Hearing Research* 42.5 (1999): 1097-1112.

28. Shimada, Michiko, et al. "Children who stutter at 3 years of age: A community-based study." *Journal of fluency disorders* 56 (2018): 45-54.

29. Leech, Kathryn A., et al. "Preliminary evidence that growth in productive language differentiates childhood stuttering persistence and recovery." *Journal of Speech, Language, and Hearing Research* 60.11 (2017): 3097-3109.

30. Finn, Patrick, Rachel Howard, and Rachel Kubala. "Unassisted recovery from stuttering: Self-perceptions of current speech behavior, attitudes, and feelings." *Journal of fluency disorders* 30.4 (2005): 281-305.

31. Shahed, Joohi, and Joseph Jankovic. "Re-emergence of childhood stuttering in Parkinson's disease: A hypothesis." *Movement Disorders: Official Journal of the Movement Disorder Society* 16.1 (2001): 114-118.

32. Plexico, Laura W., and Embry Burrus. "Coping with a child who stutters: A phenomenological analysis." *Journal of Fluency Disorders* 37.4 (2012): 275-288.

33. Adams, Martin R. "The demands and capacities model I: Theoretical elaborations." *Journal of Fluency Disorders* 15.3 (1990): 135-141.

34. Onslow, Mark, Ross G. Menzies, and Ann Packman. "An operant intervention for early stuttering: The development of the Lidcombe program." *Behavior modification* 25.1 (2001): 116-139.

35. de Sonneville-Koedoot, Caroline, et al. "Direct versus indirect treatment for preschool children who stutter: The RESTART randomized trial." *PloS one* 10.7 (2015): e0133758.

36. Franken, M. C., Koenraads, S., Stipdonk, L. (2022, May 27-29). *Long-term outcomes of the RESTART-trial comparing RESTART-DCM based treatment and the Lidcombe Program* [Conference presentation]. Joint World Congress on Stuttering and Cluttering 2022, Montreal, Canada.

37. Kalinowski, Joseph, et al. "Is it possible for speech therapy to improve upon natural recovery rates in children who stutter?" *International journal of language & communication disorders* 40.3 (2005): 349-358.

38. Chang, Soo-Eun, et al. "Functional and neuroanatomical bases of developmental stuttering: current insights." *The Neuroscientist* 25.6 (2019): 566-582.

39. Xuan, Yun, et al. "Resting-state brain activity in adult males who stutter." *PloS one* 7.1 (2012): e30570.

40. Civier, Oren, et al. "Computational modeling of stuttering caused by impairments in a basal ganglia thalamo-cortical circuit involved in syllable selection and initiation." *Brain and language* 126.3 (2013): 263-278.

41. Salmelin, R., et al. "Single word reading in developmental stutterers and fluent speakers." *Brain* 123.6 (2000): 1184-1202.

42. Civier, Oren, Stephen M. Tasko, and Frank H. Guenther. "Overreliance on auditory feedback may lead to sound/syllable repetitions: simulations of stuttering and fluency-inducing conditions with a neural model of speech production." *Journal of fluency disorders* 35.3 (2010): 246-279.

43. Smith, Anne, and Lisa Goffman. "Stability and patterning of speech movement sequences in children and adults." *Journal of Speech, Language, and Hearing Research* 41.1 (1998): 18-30.

44. Kleinow, Jennifer, and Anne Smith. "Influences of length and syntactic complexity on the speech motor stability of the fluent speech of adults who stutter." *Journal of speech, language, and hearing research* 43.2 (2000): 548-559.

45. Max, Ludo, Anthony J. Caruso, and Vincent L. Gracco. "Kinematic analyses of speech, orofacial nonspeech, and finger movements in stuttering and nonstuttering adults." (2003).

46. Kemerdere, Rahsan, et al. "Role of the left frontal aslant tract in stuttering: a brain stimulation and tractographic study." *Journal of neurology* 263 (2016): 157-167.

47. Etchell, Andrew C., Blake W. Johnson, and Paul F. Sowman. "Behavioral and multimodal neuroimaging evidence for a deficit in brain timing networks in stuttering: a hypothesis and theory." *Frontiers in human neuroscience* 8 (2014): 467.

48. Etchell, Andrew C., Blake W. Johnson, and Paul F. Sowman. "Beta oscillations, timing, and stuttering." *Frontiers in human neuroscience* 8 (2015): 1036.

49. Saltuklaroglu, Tim, Hans-Leo Teulings, and Mary Robbins. "Differential levels of speech and manual dysfluency in adults who stutter during simultaneous drawing and speaking tasks." *Human Movement Science* 28.5 (2009): 643-654.

50. Mersov, Anna-Maria, et al. "Sensorimotor oscillations prior to speech onset reflect altered motor networks in adults who stutter." *Frontiers in human neuroscience* 10 (2016): 443.

51. Salmelin, R., et al. "Functional organization of the auditory cortex is different in stutterers and fluent speakers." *Neuroreport* 9.10 (1998): 2225-2229.

52. Kikuchi, Yoshikazu, et al. "Spatiotemporal signatures of an abnormal auditory system in stuttering." *Neuroimage* 55.3 (2011): 891-899.

53. Gattie, Max, Elena VM Lieven, and Karolina Kluk. "Weak Vestibular Response in Persistent Developmental Stuttering." *Frontiers in Integrative Neuroscience* (2021): 18.

54. Max, Ludo, and Ayoub Daliri. "Limited pre-speech auditory modulation in individuals who stutter: Data and hypotheses." *Journal of Speech, Language, and Hearing Research* 62.8S (2019): 3071-3084.

55. Corbera, Sílvia, et al. "Abnormal speech sound representation in persistent developmental stuttering." *Neurology* 65.8 (2005): 1246-1252.

56. Cai, Shanqing, et al. "Weak responses to auditory feedback perturbation during articulation in persons who stutter: evidence for abnormal auditory-motor transformation." *PloS one* 7.7 (2012): e41830.

57. Cai, Shanqing, et al. "Impaired timing adjustments in response to time-varying auditory perturbation during connected speech production in persons who stutter." *Brain and language* 129 (2014): 24-29.

58. Kell, Christian A., et al. "How the brain repairs stuttering." *Brain* 132.10 (2009): 2747-2760.

59. De Nil, Luc F., et al. "A positron emission tomography study of short-and long-term treatment effects on functional brain activation in adults who stutter." *Journal of fluency disorders* 28.4 (2003): 357-380.

60. Neumann, Katrin, et al. "Assisted and unassisted recession of functional anomalies associated with dysprosody in adults who stutter." *Journal of fluency disorders* 55 (2018): 120-134.

61. Kell, Christian A., et al. "Speaking-related changes in cortical functional connectivity associated with assisted and spontaneous recovery from developmental stuttering." *Journal of Fluency Disorders* 55 (2018): 135-144.

62. Giraud, Anne-Lise, et al. "Severity of dysfluency correlates with basal ganglia activity in persistent developmental stuttering." *Brain and language* 104.2 (2008): 190-199.

63. Webster, R. L. (1975). The Precision Fluency Shaping Program: Speech Reconstruction for Stutterers, Volumes I and II, Roanoke, Virginia: Communications Development Corporation.

64. Blood, Gordon W. "A behavioral-cognitive therapy program for adults who stutter: Computers and counseling." *Journal of Communication Disorders* 28.2 (1995): 165-180.

65. Doidge, Norman. *The brain that changes itself: Stories of personal triumph from the frontiers of brain science.* Penguin, 2007.

66. Brady, John Paul. "Metronome-conditioned speech retraining for stuttering." *Behavior therapy* 2.2 (1971): 129-150.

67. Toyomura, Akira, Tetsunoshin Fujii, and Shinya Kuriki. "Effect of an 8-week practice of externally triggered speech on basal ganglia activity of stuttering and fluent speakers." *Neuroimage* 109 (2015): 458-468.

68. Toyomura, Akira, Midori Shibata, and Shinya Kuriki. "Self-paced and externally triggered rhythmical lower limb movements: a functional MRI study." *Neuroscience Letters* 516.1 (2012): 39-44.

69. Lu, Chunming, et al. "Neural anomaly and reorganization in speakers who stutter: a short-term intervention study." *Neurology* 79.7 (2012): 625-632.

70. Lu, Chunming, et al. "Reorganization of brain function after a short-term behavioral intervention for stuttering." *Brain and language* 168 (2017): 12-22.

71. Menzies, Ross G., et al. "An experimental clinical trial of a cognitive-behavior therapy package for chronic stuttering." (2008).

72. Iverach, Lisa, et al. "The relationship between mental health disorders and treatment outcomes among adults who stutter." *Journal of fluency disorders* 34.1 (2009): 29-43.

73. Miyashiro, Daiki, et al. "Altered auditory feedback perception following an 8-week mindfulness meditation practice." *International Journal of Psychophysiology* 138 (2019): 38-46.

74. Plexico, Laura, Walter H. Manning, and Anthony DiLollo. "A phenomenological understanding of successful stuttering management." *Journal of fluency disorders* 30.1 (2005): 1-22.

75. Anderson, Tracy K., and Susan Felsenfeld. "A thematic analysis of late recovery from stuttering." (2003).

76. Plexico, Laura, Walter H. Manning, and Heidi Levitt. "Coping responses by adults who stutter: Part II. Approaching the problem and achieving agency." *Journal of fluency disorders* 34.2 (2009): 108-126.

Limitations of the Lidcombe Program and the Australian Stuttering Research Centre

The Lidcombe Program is one of several treatment programs designed and offered by the self-anointed Australian Stuttering Research Centre (ASRC). While the ASRC is ostensibly a respected academic department – they have published hundreds of studies in academic journals, mostly on the speech therapy programs they devised and upon which their reputation is built – the ASRC operates more like a business than an impartial research organization.

Over the past three decades, nearly every study testing the efficacy of the ASRC's programs was conducted by the ASRC itself, without disclaimers addressing this obvious conflict of interest. While a potential conflict of interest does not necessarily lead to biased research, the ASRC is also guilty of repeated methodological errors that always seem to fall in its favor: It over-estimates positive results and either ignores or presents mitigating theories when faced with results that strongly suggest inefficacy. The ASRC then references its own studies in marketing material and academic publications as if they were conducted by an independent third-party. These circular references inflate the surface-level credibility of these studies by giving the appearance of a scientific consensus, all while obscuring the true source of the information. While this pattern holds true for all of the ASRC's treatment offerings – Westmead Program, Oakville Program, and Camperdown Program – my focus here is on the Lidcombe Program, a treatment for stuttering children.

Given the consistency and durability of these errors, as well as the ASRC's persistence in the face of criticism, I believe it is highly unlikely that these errors come from harmless mistakes; I believe this is deliberate corruption of peer-reviewed academic research. I feel it's important to add this context because most parents know next-to-nothing about stuttering when it first appears in their child, making them vulnerable to a well-organized institution that claims to have an effective remedy. And while speech therapists may read that Lidcombe has been shown to be efficacious in research, they probably do not know that the overwhelming majority of those were studies were conducted by the same people who stand to benefit from declaring the program efficacious.

Control, Persistence, and Relapse

Children who begin stuttering are capable of recovering to perfect, effortless fluency, and this recovery correlates with observable neurological changes. In fact, the vast majority of children who stutter – whether treated clinically or not – will experience this recovery. Those children who persist in stuttering, however, will have the proclivity to block for the rest of their lives. These are straightforward concepts that – outside a few fringe theories – have near-universal consensus. One would expect that the ASRC, an organization that is dedicated to stuttering treatment, would understand these concepts, but that is not the case.

While ASRC studies typically include self-laudatory refrains about the Lidcombe Program, the ASRC's leaders do not clearly state how they conceptualize success. When the ASRC claims that its program can "control" a childhood stutter,[15,16,22] one would assume that means recovery and the cessation of stuttering. However, the language of its studies – in ways that would impress a lawyer – do not *directly* state that the program causes children to recover at an increased rate. In fact, the concepts of recovery and persistence are not even mentioned in the 2021 Lidcombe Program treatment guide.[23]

Only deep in their academic publications, and usually only when pressed by outside criticism, does the ASRC state that Lidcombe is not a cure for stuttering. This is because the ASRC has a wholly different theory of childhood stuttering: "[W]e have conceptualized spontaneous recovery – from our clinical perspective – as a *management strategy*" (Emphasis mine).[21] To their mind, recovery from stuttering – even when untreated – is the result of willful effort to be fluent, rather than the cessation of the proclivity to block. By this reasoning, a persistent-but-mostly-fluent child is functionally identical to a recovered child, which completely ignores the experience of the person speaking. That's like saying hiking through a forest is the same as tiptoeing on the edge of a cliff because both involve walking!

But recovery and persistence are genuine phenomena – as evidenced by the attendant neurological changes[2] – so the ASRC must somehow account for children who continue to stutter even after months or years of Lidcombe treatment. In studies conducted by ASRC, when a child persists in stuttering after Lidcombe treatment, it is not deemed "persistence" or considered a failure of the program; instead, it is self-servingly described as a "relapse."[8,13,15] (The proposed solution, of course, is to enroll the child in the program all over again.[24]) Compare that to the 1999 study conducted by Yairi and Ambrose – who were not investigating their own proprietary program – which found that zero of their recovered children ever experienced a regression in fluency, much less began to stutter again after recovery.[30,†]

A 1997 paper on the Lidcombe Program reported that 29% of the 79 patients from a previous study "began to stutter again in the past year."[13] It seems more likely to me that they never *stopped* stuttering. Despite the obvious persistence of stuttering in some of these children – at a rate similar to the untreated children in the Yairi and Ambrose study – the authors still delivered such self-laudatory verdicts as "the long-term outcome was found to be *excellent*," and the "study did not find any cases where *permanent relapse* had occurred" (Emphasis mine). I have yet to find a clear explanation for this idea of "permanent relapse" or how it is in any way different from what the rest of the world calls "persistence."

While these conceptions of "control" and "relapse" are highly questionable, it is undeniable that the ASRC has published false information in academic journals. In a 2001 paper that laid out the history of the Lidcombe Program, Mark Onslow – co-creator of the Lidcombe Program as well as founder and director of the ASRC – wrote that "in all of the evaluations of the program to date, not a single case of relapse has been found."[22] This is not only an incredibly generous interpretation of results, it contradicts multiple studies – like the one above – which were co-authored by Onslow himself![6,7,8]

The Crusade Against Natural Recovery

Thoughtful, unbiased research on medical interventions seeks to find the exact proportion of positive

---

† A 1999 ASRC paper further muddied the boundaries between natural recovery and its own clinical outcomes by stating "Natural recovery is capable of controlling stuttering for long periods."

outcomes that can be attributed to treatment and to distinguish them from the positive outcomes that would have occurred without treatment. For a treatment program to be considered effective at treating childhood stuttering, it would have to outperform the well-documented phenomenon of untreated recovery.

Recall that in the 2018 Shimada study, 84.8% of children who were stuttering on their third birthday had recovered in the six months that followed, without receiving treatment.[28] In the 1999 Yairi and Ambrose study, 74% of the children recovered, also without treatment.[29] In order for Lidcombe to be considered an effective treatment, it needs to clearly improve upon these rates of untreated recovery.[†] The ASRC, however, has historically downplayed the prevalence of untreated recovery[21] – which, of course, would increase the apparent effectiveness of its program.[‡]

The ASRC has long suggested a significantly lower estimate of untreated recovery, based on the idea that any parental acknowledgment of the stutter means a child's

---

[†] While ASRC studies conducted before 1999 would not have access to the full results of the Yairi and Ambrose longitudinal study, a 1996 in-progress paper by Yairi and Ambrose reported 62% recovery rate for untreated children. Furthermore, the phenomenon of untreated recovery has been known since at least 1938; it is only the exact figure that has been debated and refined.

[‡] In a 2019 paper, Onslow grossly misrepresented the prevalence of natural recovery by stating "The chance of natural recovery 18 months after onset appears to be less than 10%." While it is true that only 10% of Yairi and Ambrose's children had recovered by 18 months post-onset, recovery peaked between months 12-30 for the females and months 24-36 for the males. In addition, a 1997 paper by Patrick Finn found the average and median recovery time to be 22 months. Onslow's sleight-of-hand here is akin to saying a college has a poor graduation rate because only 10% of its students complete a four-year degree in less than three years.

recovery was not "natural." Nor, to their view, did the children from the Yairi and Ambrose study experience untreated recovery, because their parents were given advice during a single counseling session.[26] This is ironic, as Yairi and Ambrose pointed out, because through this claim, the ASRC inadvertently implied that a single parental counseling session was as effective as twenty hours of the Lidcombe Program![31]

In a series of articles in the late 1990s, the ASRC aggressively criticized research on untreated recovery conducted by Yairi, Ambrose and their collaborator Richard Curlee. ASRC director Mark Onslow and his co-authors accused Yairi, Ambrose and Curlee of having insufficient data to state "that children who are reported to have recovered spontaneously are entirely and permanently stutter-free." He concluded that the three authors did not find scientific data showing that even a single child had completely recovered from stuttering without treatment. Onslow and his co-authors then haughtily suggested Yairi, Ambrose and Curlee could learn to collect more rigorous data by following his own example.[20,26]

Yairi, Ambrose and Curlee penned responses defending the rigor of their work while pointing out the paucity of data used by Onslow compared to the confidence of his assertions. In uncharacteristically strong language for an academic journal, the three researchers methodically pointed out Onslow et al.'s blatant misrepresentation of their work as well as the methodological issues, sparse data collection, and hypocritical nature behind the ASRC's accusations. They also pointedly noted that, unlike their accusers, they "do not have a motive to demonstrate a particular outcome" in their work.[4,31]

It is absurd to me that Onslow and company would launch this criticism at Yairi, Ambrose and Curlee – who did not reference Lidcombe or any other treatment program in their studies – when the ASRC drew self-serving conclusions from significantly weaker data. To me, the ASRC's criticisms seem to be an attempt to undermine research that showed a high incidence of untreated recovery because those results would lead to less demand for the ASRC's treatment program.

In a similar vein, Onslow published a criticism of the 2015 RESTART study that directly compared the effectiveness of Lidcombe and the Demands and Capacities Model (DCM).[5,23] His critique was a bit strange, considering that he believed the clinicians in that study may have been biased towards DCM because they had more experience with that program.† However, his record demonstrates that he has no concerns about the potential bias of ASRC figures investigating Lidcombe, where there are direct professional (and likely financial) attachments.[1,6,7,8,9,10,12,13,14,15,16,17,19,21,22,29] He also lamented that RESTART did not include an untreated cohort, which is odd considering that he repeatedly stated in his own studies that it is unethical to not treat stuttering children.[17] (I have long suspected that Onslow's insistence that it is unethical to use untreated controls is simply a justification to avoid directly comparing Lidcombe against lack of treatment.)

I think the true motivation behind the ASRC's critique of RESTART stems from the fact that the Lidcombe cohort returned near-identical results as the cohort of its philosophical rival, the Demands and Capacities Model.

---

† Onslow took the opposite tack when results were first presented at an academic conference, suggesting that the DCM therapists may have been delivering Lidcombe contingencies.

And, like a business, the ASRC wanted to be seen as having a superior "product" compared to its competitors.

For anyone who is curious, unconvinced, or has a serious stake in the matter, I recommend reading the handful of articles in these exchanges. The power of Yairi, Ambrose, and Curlee's writing compared to the hollow claims of Onslow and company are far more convincing than my commentary.[4,20,26,31]

Failure of the Contingencies

The core theory of the Lidcombe Program is that childhood stuttering is "responsive" to *operant conditioning*, the system of rewards and punishments made famous by B.F. Skinner's experiments in training pigeons. In Lidcombe, this conditioning is applied through the program's trademark *contingencies*, or how parents and clinicians are taught to respond to a child's speech. While never drawing a causal link from the supposed-success of the Lidcombe Program and the contingencies, Onslow and the ASRC have suggested for decades that, for some as-yet-undiscovered reason, they are the key causal factor.[8,10,16,17,19]

As far back as 2005, journal reviewers raised concerns that the ASRC was making this claim without directly testing the contingencies.[26] However, the first study to seriously investigate the contingencies was not published until 2015, twenty-five years after the first Lidcombe study was published.[6] If the contingencies were as effective as advertised, these studies would likely have turned out much differently.

The first study, conducted by a group of ASRC figures including Onslow,[3,25] investigated what would happen if one of the contingencies – the "parental request for self-correction" – was removed from the treatment program. This contingency was assumed to be particularly effective because it pointed out the undesirable behavior – stuttering – and instructed the child to perform the correct behavior: fluency. This is perfectly in tune with behaviorist theory, which states that undesirable behavioral patterns should be unlearned and replaced by desirable ones. However, the children in the study's limited version of Lidcombe showed identical improvements in fluency to the children in the regular Lidcombe Program. The obvious interpretation of these results is that this contingency had no effect on the children's fluency; however, the authors instead suggested that its beneficial aspects may have been balanced out by the children having a negative emotional response to criticism.[6] (Even though a 1997 paper by Onslow and other ASRC figures assertively defended the contingencies against criticism from the speech therapy community, writing: "we cannot see any justification for connecting that direct approach with any negative psychological impact on the child."[19])

A 2020 study by Onslow and a different selection of ASRC figures[25] went even further in its examination of Lidcombe, removing all five of the contingencies from the program. At this point, this modified version of the Lidcombe Program was like a reduced version of DCM treatment: Parents were instructed to engage with their child during conversation and give positive feedback on the child's communication without addressing the child's fluency.[7,†]

Somewhat embarrassingly for the ASRC, children in the heavily-reduced "version" of Lidcombe showed

---

† The program also included unspecified "clinical visit procedures" – which I do not believe would have meaningfully impacted recovery – and daily parental ratings of the child's fluency, which a previous ASRC study had already showed did not impact fluency.

identical improvements in fluency as the children in the full version of Lidcombe. The fluency metrics from the limited treatment group would normally have been held up by the ASRC as a success and as proof of the Lidcombe Program's singular efficacy. To me, it seems most likely that the improvements in fluency can be explained by a portion of the children in each cohort progressing towards natural recovery – exactly as was observed in the Yairi and Ambrose studies.

One might expect that, had this study been conducted by a neutral third party, the final paper would question the efficacy of Lidcombe treatment, since removing the program's core pillars had *zero effect* on outcomes. An unbiased investigator would probably raise the issue of untreated recovery; however, the published paper includes no mention of natural or untreated recovery. Or, given that the limited program resembled DCM, the authors could have compared the two – but a savvy business does not needlessly mention the competition.

Instead of re-assessing the efficacy of Lidcombe, the authors *defended* it; they concluded that there must be some other, as-yet-unknown aspect of Lidcombe that makes it so effective. In fact, despite the primary components of the treatment program being shown to be ineffective, the authors recommended that clinicians stringently follow everything laid out in the Lidcombe treatment guide!

Oddly enough, the ASRC's 2021 Lidcombe Program treatment guide still includes all five contingencies, even though its own studies found them to be non-factors.[24] These studies, which undermined thirty years of research and praise for the contingencies, were not completely ignored, though. The treatment guide audaciously states that the results from the second study "were *inconclusive*, prompting the researchers" – again, Onslow and five other members of the ASRC – "to suggest 'It is possible that verbal contingencies make some contribution to the Lidcombe Program treatment effect" (Emphasis mine).

Does this behavior suggest that the ASRC is a team of academics seeking truth through the scientific method? Is this what one would expect from a speech clinic seeking to develop an effective treatment for childhood stuttering? Or are these the actions of a business doing whatever it takes to protect its golden goose?

For all these reasons, I see the ASRC as a for-profit business masquerading as an academic department. To me, the behavior of its leaders shows a greater commitment to their own professional and financial interests than to the well-being of the children they treat and the time, effort, and money of the parents who come to them for help. The ASRC has constructed an empire with programs that do not increase the odds of resolving a childhood stutter, with research that does not hold up to independent scrutiny, and with obstinate self-assurance that its programs work.

For parents who are still interested in direct treatment for their child, there are alternative programs that administer the same philosophy just without the brand name. For those who still want to use the Lidcombe Program, the ASRC freely offers treatment guides for all of their programs on its website; these guides can be read in an hour or less. And for speech therapists, while the ASRC says that their programs are more effective when administered by speech therapists who have taken an ASRC-certified course – meaning those who paid several hundred dollars to the ASRC or an affiliate for a few hours of training – that assertion is supported only by a single, underpowered study that was conducted by (you guessed it) the ASRC.

The dozens of ASRC studies that I have read are so tainted by self-aggrandizement that I think it is best to dismiss their work altogether. Even after one learns to see through the smoke and mirrors that disguise their programs' true efficacy, there is hardly any real knowledge to be gained, because the organization's conception of childhood stuttering is fundamentally wrong; so that, as Ralph Waldo Emerson wrote, "Their every truth is not quite true. Their two is not the real two, their four not the real four; so that every word they say chagrins us, and we know not where to begin to set them right."

References

1.   Amato Maguire, Monique, et al. "Searching for Lidcombe Program mechanisms of action: Inter-turn speaker latency." *Clinical Linguistics & Phonetics* (2022): 1-13.

2.   Chow, Ho Ming, and Soo-Eun Chang. "White matter developmental trajectories associated with persistence and recovery of childhood stuttering." *Human brain mapping* 38.7 (2017): 3345-3359.

3.   "Consortium Members." *Lidcombe Program Trainers Consortium*, 24 February 2023, lidcombeprogram.org/about-lidcombe-program/consortium-members.

4.   Curlee, Richard F., and Ehud Yairi. "Early intervention with early childhood stuttering: A critical examination of the data." *American Journal of Speech-Language Pathology* 6.2 (1997): 8-18.

5.   de Sonneville-Koedoot, Caroline, et al. "Direct versus indirect treatment for preschool children who stutter: The RESTART randomized trial." *PloS one* 10.7 (2015): e0133758.

6.   Donaghy, Michelle, et al. "An investigation of the role of parental request for self-correction of stuttering in the Lidcombe Program." *International journal of speech-language pathology* 17.5 (2015): 511-517.

7.   Donaghy, Michelle, et al. "Verbal contingencies in the Lidcombe Program: A noninferiority trial." *Journal of Speech, Language, and Hearing Research* 63.10 (2020): 3419-3431.

8. Jones, Mark, et al. "Extended follow-up of a randomized controlled trial of the Lidcombe Program of Early Stuttering Intervention." *International Journal of Language & Communication Disorders* 43.6 (2008): 649-661.

9. Jones, Mark, et al. "Randomised controlled trial of the Lidcombe programme of early stuttering intervention." *bmj* 331.7518 (2005): 659.

10. Harrison, Elisabeth, Mark Onslow, and Ross Menzies. "Dismantling the Lidcombe Program of early stuttering intervention: Verbal contingencies for stuttering and clinical measurement." *International Journal of Language & Communication Disorders* 39.2 (2004): 257-267.

11. Finn, Patrick, et al. "Children recovered from stuttering without formal treatment: Perceptual assessment of speech normalcy." *Journal of Speech, Language, and Hearing Research* 40.4 (1997): 867-876.

12. Lincoln, Michelle, et al. "A clinical trial of an operant treatment for school-age children who stutter." *American Journal of Speech-Language Pathology* 5.2 (1996): 73-85.

13. Lincoln, Michelle A., and Mark Onslow. "Long-term outcome of early intervention for stuttering." *American Journal of Speech-Language Pathology* 6.1 (1997): 51-58.

14. O'Brian, Sue, et al. "Effectiveness of the Lidcombe Program for early stuttering in Australian community clinics." *International Journal of Speech-Language Pathology* 15.6 (2013): 593-603.

15. Onslow, Mark, Leanne Costa, and Stephen Rue. "Direct early intervention with stuttering: Some preliminary data." *Journal of Speech and Hearing Disorders* 55.3 (1990): 405-416.

16. Onslow, Mark. "Choosing a treatment procedure for early stuttering: Issues and future directions." *Journal of Speech, Language, and Hearing Research* 35.5 (1992): 983-993.

17. Onslow, Mark, Cheryl Andrews, and Michelle Lincoln. "A control/experimental trial of an operant treatment for early stuttering." *Journal of Speech, Language, and Hearing Research* 37.6 (1994): 1244-1259.

18. Onslow, Mark, Sue O'Brian, and Elisabeth Harrison. "The Lidcombe Programme: Maverick or Not?." *European journal of disorders of communication* 32.2 (1997): 261-266.

19. Onslow, Mark, Sue O'Brian, and Elisabeth Harrison. "The Lidcombe Programme of early stuttering intervention: methods and issues." *European Journal of Disorders of Communication* 32 (1997): 250.

20. Onslow, Mark, and Ann Packman. "Treatment recovery and spontaneous recovery from early stuttering: The need for consistent methods in collecting and interpreting data." *Journal of Speech, Language, and Hearing Research* 42.2 (1999): 398-402.

21. Onslow, Mark, and Ann Packman. "The Lidcombe Programme and natural recovery: Potential choices of initial management strategies for early stuttering." *Advances in Speech Language Pathology* 1.2 (1999): 113-121.

22. Onslow, Mark, Ross G. Menzies, and Ann Packman. "An operant intervention for early stuttering: The development of the Lidcombe program." *Behavior modification* 25.1 (2001): 116-139.

23. Onslow, Mark, and Robyn Lowe. "After the RESTART trial: Six guidelines for clinical trials of early stuttering intervention." *International Journal of Language & Communication Disorders* 54.4 (2019): 517-528.

24. Onslow, Mark, et al. "The Lidcombe program treatment guide." *Lidcombe program trainers consortium* (2021).

25. "Our Team." *University of Technology Sydney*, 24 February 2023, uts.edu.au/research/australian-stuttering-research-centre/about-asrc/our-team.

26. Packman, Ann, and Mark Onslow. "What is the take-home message from Curlee and Yairi?" *American Journal of Speech-Language Pathology* 7.3 (1998): 5-9.

27. Reitzes, Peter, host. "What is New and Exciting in Stuttering." *StutterTalk*, episode 703, 31 January 2021. https://stuttertalk.com/what-is-new-and-exciting-in-stuttering-ep-703.

28. Shimada, Michiko, et al. "Children who stutter at 3 years of age: A community-based study." *Journal of fluency disorders* 56 (2018): 45-54.

29. Woods, Sarah, et al. "Psychological impact of the Lidcombe Program of early stuttering intervention." *International Journal of Language & Communication Disorders* 37.1 (2002): 31-40.

30. Yairi, Ehud, and Nicoline Grinager Ambrose. "Early childhood stuttering I: Persistency and recovery rates." *Journal of Speech, Language, and Hearing Research* 42.5 (1999): 1097-1112.

31. Yairi, Ehud, and Nicoline Ambrose. "Spontaneous recovery and clinical trials research in early childhood stuttering: A response to Onslow and Packman (1999)." *Journal of Speech, Language, and Hearing Research* 42.2 (1999): 402-409.

32. Yairi, Ehud, and Nicoline Ambrose. "Epidemiology of stuttering: 21st century advances." *Journal of fluency disorders* 38.2 (2013): 66-87.